D0966439

Getting
Close

Getting Close

Close

*A Lover's Guide
to Embracing Fantasy and Heightening
Sexual Connection*

Barbara Keesling, Ph.D.

HarperCollins*Publishers*

Designed by Elina D. Nudelman

ISBN 0–06–017587–7

Contents

Introduction

every woman I know wishes she had a more vital connection to her sexual self, and a more vibrant connection to her loving partner. It doesn't matter if she has been married "forever" or if she is single and dating someone she has just met; it doesn't matter if she is forty-five, sixty-five, or twenty-five; it doesn't matter if she is having sex once a week or less than once a month.

What about you? Have you forgotten what it means to be filled with desire? Have you lost your erotic imagination? Is your sexual energy lacking? Has your sensual side gone unexplored for way too long? Has your love life become a comfortable, but uninspired, routine? Do you crave a profound and lasting sexual bond?

Imagine what it would feel like to have passion coursing through your veins and a sexual imagination that knows no bounds. Imagine how thrilling it would feel to be turned on by the mere sight, the smell, the touch, the voice, or even just the thought of the one you love. Imagine what it would feel like to be completely connected to the most sensual, sexual, untamed parts of you, and to be able to make this connection with your partner every time you make love. Just *imagine*.

I am a sex therapist and educator who has worked with individuals and couples for more than fifteen years. I am also a loving woman just like you. Sex is my business, but it is also my greatest passion and where my deepest commitment lies. People come to me because they want to *feel* more. This is something I hear from my clients every single day. They want to feel more passionate, more powerful, and more playful. They want to feel more sexy and more sultry, more wild and more wicked, more excited and more imaginative. They want to feel more in control and more out of control. And they want to feel more love. When these people come to me, I meet them with just one word: "connection." Connect to your sexual potential and to the sexual potential of your partnership and there are no limits to what you can feel.

The key to getting close, and to making an unforgettable sexual connection, is within your grasp right now. You are about to discover your most profound natural resource, a sleeping giant that already exists inside you just waiting to be awakened. This "secret weapon" is your erotic essence, and it will supercharge your sexual being from your fingers to your toes. I am going to help you find this essence. I am going to help you mine your passion, find your power, and develop your fullest sexual potential. And I'm going to teach you how to share this essence freely and completely with the one you love, every time you love.

Getting Close is a simple and straightforward program of erotic exercises and erotic techniques, all having one goal: to help you create a profound and lasting sexual bond. In the chapters that follow, you will learn everything you need to know about your own erotic potential, as well as the power of connecting to the one you love. You will discover special ways to touch and move, and special words that titillate and entice you. You'll discover sensuous embraces, electrifying kisses, and playful games. You will discover fantasies that inspire you, lovemaking positions that free you, and climaxes that consume you. And you will do it all in the privacy of your own home, at your own pace.

Some of the exercises and techniques are enchanting, some are intoxicating, and some are exhilarating. Some are playful, some are humorous, some are naughty, and some are downright dirty. All of them are unforgettable, and all of them have the power to transform. Whether it is the promise of a few whispered words, the passion of a lingering kiss, the excitement from skin touching skin, or the incomparable power of unbridled penetration, *Getting Close* will change the way you think and feel about sex. It will change your moods. It will change your experiences. It will change your relationships. It will change your life.

Years of professional and personal experience have taught me that there is nothing more vital and more gratifying than the richness of a close sexual connection. Sex is not just something we do on a Saturday night, it is who we are as human beings. You were built for love, and to love making love. Every single centimeter of your body—every curve, every line, every nook, every cell—is waiting to be ignited with passion, with pleasure, and with the avalanche of sensation that is *your* sexual essence. It is yours to possess and yours to share.

I have helped thousands of women feel more sexy, more sensual, more loving, more daring, more devilish, more free, more fully alive, and, most of all, more connected. Now I am going to help you. *Getting Close* will not turn you into someone you are not. It will open doors and help you step through those doors to become who you *are*—to experience your fullest, sexiest, most sensual self in an atmosphere of safety, trust, understanding, and acceptance. In my many years as a sex therapist and, before that, as a sex surrogate (a sex surrogate, or sexual surrogate partner, is a substitute partner who works directly with single people who are undergoing sex therapy), I have learned that any woman's sex life can change quickly and dramatically when she is introduced to a few simple new concepts. This book is that introduction.

GETTING CLOSE IS A THREE-STEP PROCESS

Heightening your sexual connection is a process, and I have devised a simple three-step system that will, accordingly, be laid out in this book. Sexual connection depends on sexual energy— the energy of anticipation, the energy of desire, the energy of arousal, the energy of contact, the energy of stimulation, and the energy of climax— and Part One (Level I) of this book is a step-by-step guide to finding that energy. Different chapters will explore new ways to touch, to breathe, to explore, to move, to play—even to play with food—as you fully experience the erotic potential of the body and the myriad sensations it is anxious to provide.

Part Two (Level II) of this book will focus on emotional connection and its erotic payoffs. We will explore unexpressed desire, hidden fantasy, and untamed imagination. And you will experience the transforming effects of provocative settings, evocative moods, and uncensored language.

In Part Three (Level III), we will hot-wire the connection you have been developing through Parts One and Two by bringing your partner fully onboard. We'll start with erotic communication and move on to erotic play. I'll teach you how to energize your partner and bring him up to your speed. You will discover the consuming power of complete surrender. And then I will share my "private collection" of fabulous new exercises for loving couples only. Together, you and your partner will experience an unforgettable world of intimate sensations and extraordinary pleasures as you push your erotic connection to its edges.

ALWAYS TRUST YOUR OWN BASIC INSTINCTS

In the pages that follow, I have much to share with you—many exercises, many thoughts, and many suggestions. But when it comes to your sexuality, you are the expert and you are the boss. Part of being "connected" is being able to feel what is best for you, and when it is best for you. When people visit me at my office, I have the opportunity to gather a lot more information

and be more aggressive with my guidance. But I
don't know you well enough, and I can't know
you well enough. So I trust you, and I need *you*
to trust you.

You must decide what feels good and what
feels "off." You must decide what feels too fast
and what feels too slow. You must decide what
you are ready for now, and what you may need
some time to build up to. You set the pace. You
set the intensity. You make the decisions. And
you get to say *no* wherever it suits you. Trust that
no matter what I recommend, your way of han-
dling all this material is going to be the way that
is best for you. And never try to push beyond
your emotional limits.

We all have different histories and no program
of any kind is going to be "one size fits all," but
everything in this book is meant to be *fun*. It's
normal to feel silly during some of the exercises
and it's normal to feel a little awkward with
something new, but if you start feeling unpleas-
ant or disturbing feelings, please stop what you
are doing immediately and seek help from the
appropriate quarters. A voice from inside is
telling you that you may be treading on some
difficult emotional and/or sexual material. Lots
of sound professional help is available to help
you sort this out.

TALKING TO YOUR PARTNER ABOUT
GETTING CLOSE

A wise woman once said, "A high tide lifts all boats." Tend to yourself in an attentive and loving way, and watch as your new level of self-care begins to work its magic in the relationship with the one you love. This is so true. And it is something your partner is about to discover. But a little partner preparation can go a very long way, too.

If you are in a committed relationship, I encourage you to share with your partner the bare bones of the home-study course you are embarking on. It doesn't have to be today, and it doesn't have to be this week, but it should be fairly soon. The last thing you want to have happen is to arouse suspicion or cause hurt feelings stemming from any new behaviors that may spill over into your day-to-day contact with your mate. You may want to show your partner this book and explain that you are currently at the stage where all of the exercises are practiced alone, but that later on, you hope he will join you in the exercises designed for loving couples.

Be sure to make it clear that your goal is to feel and be *closer* to him and that his patience and support at this stage are important to you and greatly appreciated. Your interest, enthusiasm, and honesty may give him a few good ideas of his own.

GETTING CLOSE STARTS WITH
SHIFTING GEARS

We're almost ready to begin. But first, I need to give you the single best piece of advice I have ever received about sexual pleasure, and I hope that you take it to heart: GREAT SEX STARTS THE MOMENT YOU SLOW DOWN. No matter what it is you are doing—getting dressed or undressed, kissing, caressing, massaging, sucking, licking, playing, humping, pumping, even masturbating—*everything* feels better when you slow it down.

Sexually speaking, most of us are doing everything way too fast. We're always cutting to the chase. We're racing to undress, racing to start screwing, racing to climax, racing to get dressed again, and racing out the door. We act as though all we want to do is get sex over with quickly. We try to make up for sensitivity with speed. And all we get is forgettable sex.

When you eat too fast, you can't taste your food. It isn't any different with sex. Believe this message and take it to heart and your sex will improve overnight. Before you do a single exercise in this book, before you even turn the page, slow everything down and start to feel the difference. Every time you touch your partner, and every time you touch yourself, cut your speed in half. Then cut it in half again.

Then cut it in half again. Now watch your pleasure multiply.

I will repeat this advice throughout the book, and you'll probably get tired of hearing it. But you'll never get tired of the results you will feel by simply slowing down.

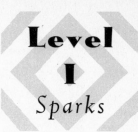

Level I
Sparks

*We're on a mission to build a roaring bonfire
inside you. But all great fires start with a few well-
placed sparks (just ask Mrs. O'Leary!). In this first
section we are going to slowly but surely start finding
the sparks that are necessary to ignite the fire of sexual energy within you—the energy that will fuel your
close connection. They are there and they are waiting.*

*Some of the sparks that you need are waiting right
now at the surface of your skin. Others are waiting
just below the surface of your body in your muscles
and tissues. Some are in your breath. Some are in the
recesses of your mind. And a few are waiting in
places that might surprise you, like in your neighbor-
hood adult toy store. We're going to visit all these
places by the time we've finished Level I.*

1

Beginning

Change begins when you make a conscious decision to start doing things differently. The mind takes the first steps. The body follows. And soon you have arrived at a very different place. By seeking out a book such as this, and having the courage to begin reading it, you have already made the conscious decision to start getting closer to the man in your life. But how will it happen? How long will it take? What will it feel like? Will it be worth the work? You may be asking yourself some, if not all, of these questions right now.

Resist the temptation to flip through all of the pages. Resist the temptation to read the end. Sit, instead, for a moment with yourself and your thoughts. And let yourself get genuinely excited about the changes that are going to begin. Now try to do something you may not do very often: Try to think about just *you*.

GETTING CLOSE:
THE FIRST SURPRISING STEP

Most women are always anxious to discover new ways to please their partners; they are ready to try almost anything or do almost anything that will bring them closer. But few can imagine that building a closer sexual connection with a man starts on the *inside,* with you. And even fewer can imagine that the best thing you can "do" for him right now is to do everything you can for *you* right now.

It would be virtually impossible to create a close sexual connection with a partner without first creating one with yourself. This is a basic fact of our sexual lives. And as I am saying this you are probably nodding your head in agreement. Yet so many books and articles seem to miss this point completely; so often, we as women miss this point completely. Instead, we worry about "him." What turns him on? What turns him off? What does he need? What does he want? What will set him on fire?

Now don't get me wrong. All of this is very important. Ultimately, it is crucial. But it isn't the place to begin, because it isn't the place where you are going to find your power. You are going to find your power by looking in the mirror. And you've got a lot of power to find. You need to meet Venus, the goddess inside you, before you meet your man. What turns you on? What turns you off? What do you need? What do you want? What will set *you* on fire? *These* are the questions we need to answer first. These are the questions that should be foremost in your mind. And before you begin a single exercise in this book, I want you to begin formulating some answers. This is the very first step you need to take. Trust me when I tell you that everything you wish for yourself and your partner will develop naturally from there.

So, as your exercises begin in this first chapter, you will notice that I am keeping your partner out of the mix. He will be part of this soon enough, and you will both be glad that you waited. My guess is that many of you are breathing a big sigh of relief right now to learn that you will have ample time to experiment and explore on your own before you're asked to get your partner involved. In my private therapy sessions, I always focus on the individual first. Even when I am seeing a couple together, much of the "homework" that I give them involves exercises to do alone; these "solo flights," so to speak, are often crucial to the success of later "duets." In this book we will begin with some of these very same exercises. Then, when it is time, we will invite your partner in. Sometimes you need to take a few steps back before you can go forward, and this is clearly one of those times. A few steps back into you, into a private place where you can be immersed in your own sexuality, will soon have you racing forward with your partner.

YOUR NEXT STEP IS GETTING A JOURNAL

I strongly suggest that you buy a divided, spiral notebook and keep a journal of your thoughts, experiences, and feelings as we progress up the path to an unforgettable sexual connection. Use your journal as the place to complete the written exercises you will come across in this book (instead of writing directly in the book). Use it also as a place to reflect on the many new and exciting sensations that you will be enjoying as you complete each exercise. A journal will allow you to mark your progress as you move toward a fuller and richer experience of your deepest sexual self. It will also help make each new experience linger. And it will help refresh and recharge your erotic memory many months, or even years, from now. (You may choose to keep your exercises in the front section and your thoughts and feelings in the back, or vice versa—whatever is most comfortable for you is the way to go.)

Obviously, it is all-important that you can write with the confidence of knowing that your journal will be free from prying eyes. If you live with a lover or husband to whom you can simply explain that what it contains is private and should not be read, fantastic (although I still would not leave it just lying around). If, on the other hand, you have children, roommates, or just an especially curious mate, you should definitely consider taking greater precautions. Perhaps you have a desk drawer that locks; or you could consider keeping it under the mattress, or, if you have to, even destroying the pages after you have written them. But the important thing is to write, and to write freely. Miraculous things can happen when you put pen to paper—I see it happen all the time. Please don't rob yourself of this gift and very important tool just because it takes a little extra effort.

GETTING CLOSE MEANS CLEANING HOUSE

Getting close to your partner means getting in touch with your thoughts and feelings about your own sexuality and female sexuality in general. We are, for example, all familiar with the jokes that get bandied about around the time a male adolescent enters puberty: "You keep that up and you'll go blind" or, "Keep doing that and it'll fall off." Charming little phrases they're not, but we know them and we laugh about them.

Now try to name *one* common phrase or joke that refers to something equally natural and commonplace: female adolescent masturbation. Are you drawing a blank? Are you catching my drift? For young boys the message is, "It might not be approved of, but it's expected." For young girls the message is, "Masturbation is taboo; you don't talk about it, and you don't even joke about it."

This is just one message that has shaped your sexual connectedness, but there are so many others. The truth is that by the time you have found your way to this book, you have received and internalized *thousands upon thousands* of messages about sex and sexuality. Messages about masturbation, messages about your body, messages about intercourse, messages about orgasm, messages about pleasure. On and on it goes. We need to get to some of those messages before we go any farther; we need to clean house. And that is the purpose of this very first exercise.

"Connection" Exercise #1: Writing Yourself Clear
Open your notebook. In this first exercise, you're going to explore some of the beliefs and thoughts you hold about sex and sexuality and about your body and femininity. This is an excellent exercise for determining where you currently are in regard to many of the issues we will be dealing with in

this book. You can be as lenghty or as brief as you like in your responses. The idea is to get as many of these old mes- sages out in the open where you can take as close a look at them as possible. Dig deep and leave no stone unturned. We're cleaning house, so it's time to lift the rug and move the chest of drawers to get at those dust bunnies.

At the top of the page, write:
1. AS A YOUNG GIRL, THE MESSAGES I RECEIVED ABOUT SEX WERE . . .

At the top of the next page, write:
2. AS A YOUNG GIRL, THE MESSAGES I RECEIVED ABOUT MY BODY WERE . . .

At the top of the next page, write:
3. AS A YOUNG GIRL, THE MESSAGES I RECEIVED ABOUT MASTURBATION WERE . . .

Now finish each sentence. Give yourself plenty of time and try to go into extensive detail, with illustrative exam- ples (e.g., "I remember one time when I was seven years old, my mother told me . . .", "I remember the first time I had my period, my best friend told me . . .", "I remember the first time I masturbated and I . . .", "I remember read- ing a book about sex that said . . .", "I remember the first time a boy tried to kiss me, I . . .").

Don't feel you have to complete all three questions in one sitting. This material is so very important and we want to get as much as possible out of your brain and your body and onto the paper where it can help you. If you need more than one page for each answer, take it. If you write an entire book for each one, you might need a literary agent.

Did you write a lot, or a little? Sometimes, the strongest messages we receive are the unspoken ones. So even if you didn't write much of anything, that in itself speaks volumes about the way sex was viewed in your home. Are you surprised by anything you wrote down? Sometimes we think that we know all there is to know about ourselves until we start rooting around a little bit.

Keep these pages for a day or two, and add to them as memories and recollections come up for you. HOWEVER, when you have finished the writing and finished your reflecting, it is *very* important for you to eventually destroy these three lists. Let me tell you why. Unless you are the one-in-a-million woman who was raised with a healthy, open regard toward sexual expression and your body, your lists are probably brimming over with old-wives' tales, stereotypes, and all manner of joy-killing, sex-dampening garbage that **needs to be gotten rid of!** You've held on to it for far too long. So shred them, rip them up into a million little pieces, or carefully burn them in your fireplace, but be sure to physically destroy these lists.

GETTING CLOSE MEANS SOME HEAVY BREATHING

I know what you're thinking! But that kind of heavy breathing will come later. To get started, we need to be doing a different kind of breathing that will help you get focused on you.

Before and after each exercise in this book (even the writing exercises), it's a good idea to take a series of deep, cleansing, sensual breaths. A sensual breath is a long, *slow*, deep inhalation through the nose that makes your tummy rise, and a long, slow exhalation through the mouth that makes your tummy go down. Sensual breaths are energizing and relaxing at the same time and can help center and calm you. I always visualize white, purifying light entering my body with each breath, and all tension and negativity leaving my body with each exhalation. Let's try some now.

"Connection" Exercise #2: The Sensual Breath
Lie on your back or sit comfortably. Place your hand over your abdomen. Slowly breathe in through your nose— feel your hand rising on your belly as you draw air deep into your lungs. Imagine white light filling every square inch of your body, energizing and focusing you. Feel the air caress you as it fills you. Now exhale slowly through your mouth. As you exhale, imagine all of the negativity held in any of the statements you wrote down released

and scattered to the winds. All of those oppressive and false beliefs that still live somewhere inside you have received their "pink slips," been given their walking papers . . . next! It's time for a new set of beliefs, a new way of seeing yourself and regarding your sexuality. Make room for the "new you" with each exhalation. Feel your hand go down as your belly expels the air. Take two or three more sensual breaths. Then relax and breathe normally for a few minutes. Be sure to check in with yourself. How are you feeling? When you're ready, take two or three more sensual breaths. During this second round of breathing, pause for three seconds between breathing out and breathing in. Don't pause between breathing in and breathing out; the inhalation and exhalation should flow seamlessly.

You can repeat the sensual breath cycle as many times as you feel is necessary to fully relax and recharge. Before your exercises, you will use the sensual breath to slow you down and bring you to center; after the exercises you will use it to help sensations linger and reinforce the learning process. You can also use the breath cycle throughout the day whenever you need a pick-me-up or to relieve stress. Let it become a regular part of your life; it is a wonderful companion.

And now I need to say congratulations! It may not feel as though you have done anything drastic yet. It may not feel as though you have done anything at all! But trust me when I tell you that by completing these few very simple exercises you have just taken your first giant steps toward getting close and making an unforgettable sexual connection. As we proceed to the next chapter, and actively explore the world of "touch," you will begin to understand why I say this.

2
Touching

When was the last time you touched yourself? And no, I don't mean to brush the hair out of your eyes or scratch the tip of your nose. I mean *really* touched yourself—*felt* yourself? You probably remember from high school biology class that the skin is the largest organ of the human body. Being the dedicated sex therapist that I am, I like to say that the skin is the largest *sex* organ on the body, too. When we enjoy a great lover, what is it, really, that sets him apart? Isn't it his touch? Isn't it the way he seems to know just where to brush with the back of his hand—just where to caress—just where to gently squeeze? How did he learn to do that? Practice, practice, practice—and a strong *desire*. It isn't hard to imagine a man who has slept with a lot of women but still is not a sensitive or imaginative lover, is it? In fact, we may have even *known* one or two in our time. So what sets our Don Juan apart from our Joe Blow? The desire to please and the knowledge about how to do it.

Unfortunately, it has been my experience that most women take the Joe Blow approach to themselves when it comes to self-touch and self-love. Women have been systematically taught to disown their bodies—don't ask, don't tell, and for God's sake, DON'T TOUCH! Well, ladies, all of that is about to change. You are going to learn what to touch and when to touch it. You're going to learn what turns you on the most—you are going to become experts at making yourselves feel good. Once you learn how, you will have access to this power whenever you want it. And later on you'll be able to incorporate your new expertise into lovemaking with your partner for mind-blowing results . . . but I'm getting ahead of myself.

FIRST THINGS FIRST: THE LOVING TOUCH

You can think of this chapter as Touching 101, your introduction to being touched the way you were made to be touched. In this next exercise, you are going to make your very first true *touch* connection, one of the most important building blocks for a comprehensive sexual connection. Making the touch connection means learning to focus on the sensations that are created when you *lightly* and *continuously* stroke and caress your body. From now on I'm going to refer to this very special kind of caress as "loving touch" because that's really what it is. Loving touch is not deep tissue massage and your intent is not to become sexually stimulated. It's okay if you do, but that's not our goal with loving touch. There's no pressure here; this is not a test. You are simply, and perhaps for the first time ever, going to stroke yourself all over for the sheer pleasure of it.

Things you will need:

1. *A quiet room free from distractions.*
   Unplug the phone and leave the kids with your mother if you have to, but carve out some time for yourself. Give yourself at least a full hour.

2. *Hypoallergenic massage oil or baby oil, and KY jelly.*
   Use massage oil or baby oil for your full-body loving touch but, to avoid irritation, stay with KY jelly or something comparable when caressing the genitals.

3. *Soothing music.*
   If you have a stereo or CD player in your room, put on some soothing, *lyric-free*

music. Music with lyrics might prove to be
too much of a distraction. But some gentle classical, New Age, or jazz will help
you relax and create a mood conducive to
your self-exploration.

4. A clean towel and clean hands.

"Touching" Exercise #1

*Undress. Spread your towel on a bed or other comfortable
surface where you can stretch out completely. Lie back.
Take several deep, cleansing breaths.*

*How does it feel to lie out in the nude? Do you do it
often? Sometimes? Never? Try to isolate areas where you
might be holding tension in your body and breathe into
them. Imagine the white light rushing to those areas as you
inhale and relax the muscles.*

*Pour a little of the massage oil into your hands and then
rub them together to warm it. If the oil is scented, inhale
deeply and let the aroma stir your senses.*

*Place your fingertips lightly on your body. Move your
fingers ever so slowly over the surface of your skin. Keeping
your eyes closed, pretend you have never seen a body before,
so that every inch is a new discovery. Go very slowly. Touch
your face, your eyelids, the back of your neck, your collar-
bone, your breasts, your nipples. Pay close attention to the
textures and shapes of your different body parts. If your
mind starts to wander or you feel yourself moving into judgment about your body, **slow down** and try to focus only on*

the **sensations** that are created by touching your own body in this sensuous way.

Move down your body at a slow, languorous pace. Slide a finger over your belly button. Trail your fingers between your buttocks cheeks; slowly rub between your toes. Pause for more baby oil, if you need it. Touch your thighs and behind your knees.

How are you feeling? Remember to breathe. When you are fully relaxed and only when you are ready, slowly apply some KY jelly to your vagina with your fingers. Although you may be feeling aroused, the goal is not to bring yourself to orgasm right now, but to become intimate with the way your body feels and responds to touch. Just go with the flow and let whatever happens, happen.

Slightly part your legs. Use the same slow, light touch you used over the rest of your body. Lightly stroke the hood of your clitoris. Slide it back; feel it slide forward again. Find the outer and inner lips of your vagina. Gently pull them apart, then let them go. Stroke the entryway to your vaginal canal. Just barely insert a finger into your vagina. Be aware of the texture inside your vagina and the pressure that is exerted on your finger.

Slowly, slowly glide your finger all the way in. How does the texture inside your vagina change? Touch your cervix, if you can. Your cervix will feel like a hard, round knob deep within your vagina (be careful feeling your cervix if you have long fingernails!). Let yourself become familiar with the shape and feel of your own vagina—it's as one of a kind as a snowflake, and as beautiful. Own it!

Allow yourself at least twenty minutes for the genital loving touch, but if time allows, spend as long as you like with it.

When you have completed your first full-body loving touch, let yourself bask for a few minutes in the feelings you have created for yourself. Do you feel differently than you did when you first started the loving touch? How? Take some cleansing sensual breaths. Be sure to exhale completely. Thank yourself for giving yourself this gift of time, energy, and attention, and be sure to record your experience in your journal.

AN AFFAIR TO REMEMBER

Now that you have taken your first few steps toward creating a compelling sexual connection, I think it's important to speak about the concept of having your first affair. Don't panic. I have no intention of destroying the loving relationship you already have. What I'm talking about here is having an exciting, tawdry affair with *yourself!* Let me explain.

In these early stages of forging a bond with your sexual core, you may begin to feel as though you are carrying on a clandestine affair. Your heart is beating a little faster. You're thinking about sex all the time. You're being a little secretive with your new sexual discoveries. And you have a new partner who is pretty hot—YOU! This is great. In fact, I encourage it. If the exercises I have designed in this book can help you *fall in love with yourself*, with your body, with the pleasure it can give you, and with your sexuality, I will feel I have done my job.

I am going to make what may strike you as a very radical statement—I truly believe that all women should have two sex lives: one with a partner, and one with themselves. In the same way that I think it is important to prepare a nice meal and set a place for yourself at the table when your partner is away (instead of eating over the sink!), I believe it is equally important that you care for your "sexual body" in a way that speaks of your respect and reverence for it.

In a way, this relates back to my earlier statement about women tending to disown their bodies. In these late 1990s, it is common for a woman to hold a job outside the home, for a woman to hold separate political beliefs from her partner, for a woman to own and drive her own car . . . but to not rely solely on her partner for all of her sexual validation and pleasure? For some reason, this is still a radical notion. I believe in togetherness. I believe in partnership. I believe that the emotional and spiritual fulfillment that come from sharing a life with someone you love are heaven on earth. But I also believe that the more we learn to give to *ourselves*, the more we learn to *fulfill* ourselves, the more we actually enrich our partnerships while immeasurably improving the quality of our individual lives as well.

Having a loving, gratifying affair with yourself begins by learning to touch yourself in ways that only you can. And the more ways you learn to touch, the richer the experience for you and, ultimately, for your partner as well. Which brings us to our next exercise.

THE LOVING, WET TOUCH

In this second phase of developing your sense of touch, I want you to go skinny-dipping . . . but don't panic! I recommend you do it in your very own bathtub. This will not be your ordinary bath, however. Instead of getting clean, you're going to get a little "dirty."

Believe it or not, water has played a part in some of the most stunning transformations it has been my privilege to witness in all my years as a sex therapist. One story in particular comes to mind. I was counseling a young, newly married couple who I will call Mike and Sue. The problem they were having was that Sue could not orgasm. She couldn't orgasm alone, she couldn't orgasm with Mike. She couldn't orgasm through oral sex, she couldn't orgasm through intercourse. We tried everything and nothing was working. Finally, in desperation, I suggested they just take a long sensuous bath together.

Well, the next day I received a very excited phone call. Somehow, the relaxing, buoyant nature of the water enabled Sue to get out of her head, relax into her body, and get past the last of her inhibitions. (The water also provided a constant lubricant for Mike's slippery hand.) Suffice it to say, their fingertips looked a lot like prunes for the next few days. And once Sue learned to orgasm in the bathtub, she was, within a matter of weeks, able to climax in other rooms of the house as well.

We all know how relaxing a nice hot soak can be. But you're about to discover what a completely erotic experience bathing for one can be, just by shifting your intent. Remember, you don't want to get clean, you want to get dirty. So, no rubber duckies allowed!

What you'll need:

1. *Time.*
   Again, time and privacy are the first things you need to secure for yourself in abundance. Try to allow an hour and a half for this exercise.

2. *Aromatic bath oils and bubble bath.*
   Spend just a little or spend a lot, but get something special for yourself. You *don't*

want to use your kid's Mr. Bubble for this
one!

3. *Scented candles.*
   Try to take your skinny dip at night. We
   are more conditioned to equate night-
   time with erotic possibility.

4. *Music.*
   This time, the music is very important. So
   even if it's the clock radio from your night-
   stand, find a station that's mellow and sexy;
   create a sensuous setting for yourself.

5. *Tub spa (optional, but highly desirable).*
   Do you happen to have water jets in your
   tub? If not, how about one of those
   whirlpools that attaches to the rim of your
   tub? If the answer is yes to either of those
   questions, turn it on, sister! If you
   answered no, it's not the end of the world,
   but I find that the whirlpool is extremely
   relaxing and helps you to make that connection with your sensual core even faster.

"Touching" Exercise #2
Light the candles, turn on the music, and slip into your
scented, sensual bath. Close your eyes. Take three deep sen-

sual breaths. Let all outside cares and concerns slip away for the time being; be present for yourself in this moment.

Begin your loving touch. Move your fingertips **sloooowly** over the surface of your wet skin. Keep the contact light and focus your attention only on the pleasurable sensations that are created by your touch. Take your time; there is absolutely no rush. Leave no inch of your surface skin untouched. Trace the outline of all the places where you curve in—and all of the places where you curve out. Lift your arm and slowly touch yourself from the wrist to the armpit. Stay aware of which areas respond most to being touched. Take at least thirty minutes to complete your full-body touch.

Now, begin a slow and thorough genital loving touch. Start your fingers at the most sensitive portion of your inner thighs and slowly move toward your pubic mound, then down to your clitoris. After fully exploring your clitoris, ever so slowly trail a finger or two from your clitoris down across your vulva to your anus, then back to your vulva. Go as slowly as you possibly can. Feel how the lips of your vulva part at your touch. Go ahead and slip a finger into your vagina. Although you're probably feeling pretty good right now, try not to masturbate. Just be aware of the feelings that are being created by your touch and continue with your sensory exploration. Open up your senses to the feeling of your vagina in the water. How does the water make the inside of your vagina feel? Slowly continue your "finger trail" until you reach your anus again. Let yourself feel how sensitive this opening is to the slightest touch. Run your fingers farther up the crack between your buttocks before changing directions and moving back toward your vagina. Take as much time as you need to take.

As you continue with this exercise, resist the temptation to bring yourself to orgasm. Instead, in keeping with the same manner in which it was built, let your state of arousal rise and then slowly subside, then rise again and subside again. Continue in this fashion—up and down, but never climaxing. I call this technique "peaking," and it is a highly useful tool in stoking the fires of anticipation and desire.

In the same way that a tasty morsel serves as an appetizer to awaken your hunger for a full meal, peaking serves to awaken your hunger and capacity for sexual fulfillment. Peaking puts your sensitive nerve endings "on call," so to speak, and right now, you want those nerves to stay awake and "smell the coffee" for as long as possible. So leave them begging for more, if you have to. It may be a little uncomfortable now, but I promise you, the payoff later will make it all worthwhile.·

As your state of arousal subsides each time, try to imagine how quickly you could bring yourself back to a highly aroused state from these lower "plateaus" if you touched yourself now . . . or now. You won't actually touch yourself, just visualize it for now.

Good work! You're probably starting to feel more intimate with your body and your sexual core than you have in a long time. And the good news is, we've only just begun! Remember to write down your thoughts and feelings in your sex journal when you're through. Don't forget to blow out the candles!

DEVELOPING YOUR ESP
(EXTRA-SENSUAL PERCEPTION)

Have you ever wondered why it is that when you were a teenager, just holding hands with your sweetheart was enough to make the hairs on your arms stand up and why now, even making love with your loved one does not seem to have the ability to excite you in that same electric way? It is one of the most frequently asked questions I receive from women who are interested in reinvigorating their sexual lives with their partners.

For many years I struggled with this question, both professionally and personally. The most obvious conclusion to come to would be that after a while, *everything* loses its luster once you get used to it. And that it's *impossible* to maintain the same level of excitement in a relationship that you've been in for a while compared to when it was new. But something in me has never been able to accept such a bleak scenario for long-term, loving couples.

For some of the women who came to me, it quickly became apparent that there were underlying problems, such as unexpressed anger or resent-

ment, that could be causing them to shut down
around sex. In those cases, individual and/or couples therapy is often necessary before any of the
sexual issues can be addressed.

But what about the woman who is otherwise
happy with her relationship, in love with her
mate, but whose steak has lost just about all of
its sizzle? What realistic, workable solution is
there for bringing back the passion she once felt
for her man?

After prescribing the same program of exercises to dozens of different women all suffering
from the same problem, I believe I have found a
remedy for the malaise that so many of you have
described as occurring in your sexual lives. I
believe it is possible to recharge your sexual battery, refuel your sexual engine, and reinspire
your sexual feelings by developing your extra-
sensual perception.

What is extra-sensual perception? It is the
ability to translate everyday sounds, touches,
thoughts, music, smells, and tastes into sexual
triggers. It is the ability to find sexual reminders
in what you now consider to be mundane and
common items and occurrences. If extra-
sensory perception is the sixth sense, then
extra-sensual perception is the seventh. Using
an automobile analogy, if I may (I *do* live in

California, after all), a well-developed ESP will
take you from zero to sixty, sexually speaking,
like a well-tuned Ferrari, as opposed to the gas-
efficient little compact car you're used to hous-
ing your sexual drive in.

Developing your ESP requires retraining yourself—your body, your mind, and your soul—to
think about sex *all of the time*, and to constantly
see yourself as a sexual being.

I may not be able to see you, but I definitely
heard some eyes rolling out there. "What does
she mean 'think about sex all of the time'; what
does she think we are, *teenagers*?!" By George, I
think you've got it! Exactly my point. If you want
to feel the *urgency* that a teenager feels—the *passion* that a teenager feels, the *heat* that a
teenager feels, the *lust* that a teenager feels—
then you've got to *think* like a teenager; and
teenagers think about SEX!

Developing your extra-sensual perception
means retuning your sensual "tuning fork" to a
frequency you probably haven't picked up in a
while. It really isn't hard to do; in fact, it's a lot of
fun. A well-developed ESP is bound to make you
feel more alive, more powerful, and more connected. You're going to become "Ms. Sensitive,"
sexually speaking—a woman who can "idle high"
and be capable of a quick response.

The exercises you have already completed

serve as a foundation for all of the other exercises put forth in this book, and were your first steps taken toward strengthening your ESP. Use them any time you need to reconnect with yourself or to "warm up" before having sex. But, as you might suspect, we're just getting started . . .

THE LOVING, HOVERING TOUCH

Your sensitivity training continues as we combine the techniques you learned in the first two exercises with a few new twists that will raise you off the ground and will raise your extra-sensual perception to staggering new heights. So prepare yourself as you did for "Touching" Exercise #1. Gather your oils, your music, and your towel. But this time you will also need a *blindfold*. Choose a silky scarf or a soft bandanna; even a sleep mask will do. Are you ready for some extraordinary sensual perceptions? Are you already starting to tingle? Then let's get back to work.

"Touching" Exercise #3
Undress and lie down on your towel. Tie your blindfold lightly, but securely, over your eyes. Begin the sensual breath sequence, inhaling slowly and deeply. Remember to picture the white light relaxing the spots that hold tension in your body. Exhale fully and hold your breath for three seconds at the end of each exhalation.

*Rub some oil between the palms of your hands and com-
mence your loving touch. Go as slowly as you possibly can.
Notice how the blindfold serves to heighten the eroticism of
your touch. Be creative with your touch: Use only one finger on both hands for a while, then two, then three, etc.
Extend your fingers. Now lightly move your palms over
your nipples, your face, your neck. . . . Lift your pelvis and
run your palms lightly over your buttocks; stroke your
palms over your pubic hairs, and the hood of your clitoris.*

*Now raise your palms a quarter of an inch off your skin
and let them **hover** just over your body **without making
any direct contact**. Feel the energy pulsate between the
palms of your hands and the surface of your skin.
Visualize sparks dancing between them. Ever so slowly
start moving your hands up, down, and around the surface of your body. Go slower than you've ever gone before.
Think of the palms of your hands as magnets that are
drawing the electricity from your nerve endings **beyond** the
surface of your skin. Hover over your most sensitive spots:
your nipples, your belly button, your vagina. Focus on the
sensation in your hands, then SWITCH YOUR FOCUS
to the sensation in the body part you're hovering over.
Switch your focus back to your hands. Switch again to
your body. Try this for several minutes. Breathe deeply. Be
aware of your feelings.*

Some of my clients report that their palms
start feeling itchy or warm. Others say that their
bodies feel electric. Some say the erotic tension

is so strong they can barely stand it. What about you? Are you marveling at the fact that you can feel tingly, excited, or even fully aroused *without even touching yourself*? That's a sure sign of a developing ESP.

3

Dancing

What do you think of when you hear the word "dance"? Here are some of the words that come to my mind: body, movement, rhythm, muscles, power, sexy, open, wild, crazy, free, free, free. Dancing is a metaphor for freeing the body and the spirit. It's about losing your mind (not literally, of course) and coming into your senses. And it's about giving up control. This is a metaphor I want you to embrace.

Making a mesmerizing sexual connection means getting out of your head and getting immersed in feelings and sensations. It means learning how to dance inside your erotic essence, feeling free and fully alive. And that is what this chapter is all about. To get you there I am going to ask you to dance—not figuratively, but literally. You are going to use your body to get to your feelings, to get to your energy, and to get to your wild side. It doesn't matter if you haven't danced since the Bee Gees were "Staying Alive" and the last dance step you mastered was the bump. The type of dancing I am talking about focuses zero percent on form and one hundred percent on content. And the music is about to start . . .

CLEAR THE DANCE FLOOR

This is going to be a solo performance, so choose a time when you are assured of total privacy for at least one hour (two is even better). Also, give yourself some elbow room. If you can, move a few pieces of furniture so you will have more room to maneuver. It might also be a good idea to move any free-standing vases or other breakable objets d'art to higher ground.

Change into some soft, comfortable clothing. Scour your record and/or CD collection for dance music you haven't listened to for a while. What were you dancing to in high school? The Sex Pistols? Sly and the Family Stone? Elvis? Whomever or whatever it was that used to get you going, find it. Now get ready for your first exercise. Your goal with this exercise is a very simple one: to get completely lost in the music.

"Dancing" Exercise #1: Body Rhythms

Start to play some of your favorite dance music. If you like your music loud and you can play it that way without disturbing anyone, pump up the volume and let the music surround you. Otherwise, keep the volume at a comfortable level.

*As you first listen to the music, close your eyes and let its beat seep into your bones. I want you to start **slow**, keeping your movement to a minimum at this point. You can nod your head in time with the music or tap your foot, but let the rhythm grow and build inside you in the same way that sexual excitement builds. Let the music move **you** instead of **you** moving to the music.*

Slowly let the music inspire you to more and more movement. Forget about what you look like, just make sure that your movement is organic. It should be rising up from inside you, not coming from your head where you hold a picture of what you think dancing is supposed to be. Connect with the most soulful part of yourself and express it freely. Lose yourself in the music.

FLASHDANCING FANTASIES

Do you remember the movie *Flashdance*? It's a hard one to forget. The dancing was so exciting and compelling and thoroughly sexual that every woman I know left with fantasies of finding a club where she could let herself get that wild. If you had those fantasies too (and even if you didn't), here's your chance to do some acting out. (If you've never seen *Flashdance*, go straight to your local video store right now, rent it, and watch it before we continue.)

The first thing you need to do is make sure you are wearing clothes that you can get wild in—I recommend something snug and sexy such as a leotard or short shorts. Now find some of your fastest, most rhythmic, most upbeat dancing music and get ready for the show to start.

"Dancing" Exercise #2

Start the music at a low volume. Close your eyes and let it enter your body. Feel the beat. Become the beat. After a minute or two, open your eyes and start turning up the volume. Build it slowly, feeling it strengthen as you go, until it is as loud as your ears and your neighbors can tolerate. Now cut loose.

Dance like you have never danced before. Get crazy. Lose control. Jump around like a wild woman if that's what feels appropriate to you. Or get down an all fours and sway back and forth. Do the shimmy shake, clap your hands, hoot and holler, work up a sweat! Do a few gymnastic moves, if you can. Or a series of tumbles. Free yourself down to your foundation.

Dance until you're laughing, dance until you're crying, but dance until you've touched something in yourself that you haven't felt touched in a long, long time.

GOING TO A GO-GO

In the last two exercises, you got a chance to remember how uninhibited dance can be used as a tool to tap into a deep river of energy that can revitalize every aspect of your life: your emotional life, your spiritual life, your health and well-being. And I bet you're starting to feel pretty sexy, too. Well, this was your warm-up; now you're ready for a thorough cooking. If the free and large gestures in the first dances were like an explosion, the smaller, more controlled movements in this next dance will be more like an *implosion*. It's time to go from the macro to the micro and focus specifically on rousing just your *sexual* energy.

What you will need:

1. *Clothing.*
   For this exercise you'll need a full-length mirror and something to wear that makes you feel *really* sexy. It could be your favorite teddy, a slinky black dress, or one of your lover's long-sleeved shirts rolled up to the elbows. You want to feel *super* sexy, so take off your bra and panties.

2. *Music.*
   Put on music that is *sensual* to you. I find the singer Sade's voice can instantly put

me in a very sexual frame of mind. What singer makes you think about making love? That's whose music you want to play for this next exercise.

"Dancing" Exercise #3

With your sexy outfit on, stand in front of the full-length mirror and make eye contact with yourself. Let the music very gently impel you to move. You want to dance slowly and sensuously. Move mostly from your hips. Stay in front of the mirror. Watch yourself undulate, tease, seduce.

Close your eyes and imagine you are making love. How would it feel to have your lover's penis inside you right now? How would you move if it were? Imagine that your nipples are being teased with a tongue; how would it feel? Let yourself respond. Are you moaning? Is your head thrown back with pleasure? Continue moving sensuously to the music; look yourself in the eye from time to time.

Look at how sexy and turned on you look. Feel how sexy and turned on you are. Celebrate how sexy and turned on you can get.

THE BELLE OF THE "BALL"

You have a very important dance partner who has been with you all along, but who can be shy and retiring until she has had a few lessons to learn the steps. Actually, this partner isn't a person, it's a muscle. And as far as your sex life is concerned, it is the most important muscle in your body.

It is known as the PC muscle. You and your PC muscle are the "two" it takes to tango. By faithfully practicing a few simple steps, you and your PC muscle can enjoy a lifetime together of tripping the light fantastic on the dance floor of love!

What, Where, When, and . . .

The PC muscle is an affectionate term for what is technically known as the pubococcygeal muscle group. This group of muscles cradles your pelvic organs and sweeps from your pelvic bone in the front of your body to your tailbone in the back.

A strong PC muscle contributes to your sexual pleasure in many ways. The muscle actually spasms when you have an orgasm, creating a feeling of tightness in the vagina. It makes sense then that the stronger the PC muscle, the stronger the spasm and the more intense your orgasm can be. That is reason number one for strengthening your PC muscle.

Here is reason number two: A well-developed PC muscle can grip an object—an object such as a penis (to name my favorite example) or a dildo (which we'll talk about later)—more forcefully, applying more pressure to your sensitive vaginal walls, and even your G-spot (watch out!). In plain English, this feels *really fabulous*! And if it's a penis you're gripping, it feels pretty darn good to your partner, too.

So those are two great reasons to get your PC muscle in shape. Hopefully, they're all the reasons you need. But if you need a few more, read on.

Strengthening your PC muscle is also healthy. A strong PC muscle is the best defense against incontinence in older age. And if you are in your childbearing years, not only will a fit PC muscle help you during childbirth, it will help you recover your muscle tone more quickly after pregnancy as well. We could all use that kind of help.

So here's the bottom line: If you can make the following exercise as much a daily habit as brushing your teeth and taking your vitamins, you will be doing more to take control of and enhance your sexual pleasure than anything else I could possibly recommend. How's that for an endorsement?

Pulling a Muscle from Its Shell

Has my sales pitch sold you? Are you ready for the exercises? I'm almost ready to share them. But in order to firm up your PC muscle, you must first *find* your PC muscle. And that's what we need to do right now.

Have you ever been taking a pee and then thought you heard the phone ring or your child call out for you? Do you know that muscle you squeeze to stop the flow of urination so that you can hear more clearly? *That*, dear lady, is your almighty PC muscle at work. Try to give it a little squeeze right now.

Some of us are more successful at stopping the flow than others. If you are able to stop a strong flow midstream, then your PC muscle is already in good shape. But if your attempts to interrupt the flow of urine don't even slow it down, it's an indication that your muscle needs to be toned. But no need to despair! It can be done easily and in a short amount of time; you don't even have to buy new workout clothes! The following exercises will show you how.

"Dancing" Exercise #4

Start with clean hands. Breathe deeply into your stomach and relax your abdominal muscles. While lying comfortably on your back or sitting on the toilet, insert your index finger about two inches into your vagina.

Squeeze with the muscle you use to stop the flow of urination. Keep **breathing** *while you squeeze the muscle. You may feel your finger being drawn up into your vagina, or you may feel just the faintest flutter. But if you feel pressure on your finger and you are not pressing with*

your thigh and buttock muscles, you have located your
PC. Done correctly, no one should be able to look at you
and tell you are flexing your PC muscle. It's your little
secret, your little dance.

Now that you have met your new dance partner, it is time for the two of you to learn the
steps that will waltz you into ecstasy every time
you make love.

"Dancing" Exercise #5

Take a deep, cleansing breath. Flex and hold your PC muscle for approximately two seconds. Release the hold. Let
your PC muscle completely relax before flexing again.
Make sure you're not holding your breath while you flex the
muscle. Try not to tense up; breathe normally. Repeat the
flex and hold the sequence.

During week number one, do ten repetitions at a time,
three times a day. If ten repetitions are too much for you,
start with five and work up to ten as you are able.
During week number two, add five repetitions so that
you are doing fifteen at a time. By week number three,
you will add five more repetitions for a total of twenty. It
really should take from three to six weeks to get to that
point. Trying to do too much, too fast can overwork the
muscle and make it sore. At the end of three weeks, your
PC muscle should be well toned. A slow approach is
best; so, easy does it!

DANCING MORNING, NOON, AND NIGHT

I hope that "flexing" on a daily basis will become
as automatic to you as flossing on a daily basis.
Your PC flexes can be practiced absolutely anywhere, at any time of the day. Try doing them
right around breakfast, lunch, and dinner. That
way, the meal acts as a reminder to you.

One of the truly rewarding things about this
"exercise" is that it quickly becomes an erotic
act. As your muscle strengthens, each squeeze
will trigger very alive, horny sensations, clearly
reminding you of the sexual creature you are
(let's see "feel the burn" do that!). When your
muscle gets really strong, it may even "flutter"
involuntarily from time to time, sending a sexy
chill through your sensitive body when you least
expect it. Yum.

Later on in Level I, you will receive a very
graphic demonstration of what this wonderful and
powerful muscle is capable of. But right now I just
want you to dance with your new partner. So put
your sensual music back on, put your sensual outfit (from "Dancing" Exercise #3) back on, and get
ready for your last dance of the evening.

"Dancing" Exercise #6

Listen to the music and slowly begin your sensual mirror
dance the way you did in "Dancing" Exercise #3. Once

*again, connect to the erotic energy in your body and your most natural sexual rhythms. As you seductively move to the music, start to squeeze your PC. Squeeze it rhythmically, using it to help keep the beat. Feel how it focuses you. Feel how it energizes you. Feel how it eroticizes you. Feel how it **connects** you. Feel the strength your body has found.*

It's time to take a well-deserved break so your sensual batteries can recharge. You have now had your first taste of the power and passion that live inside you. Your next taste, in the chapter that follows, is more than a mouthful. So rest, shower, and get a good night's sleep. And dream of the treats that await you.

4

Tasting

*t*his may sound a little silly to you, but when I was a young woman I was practically addicted to my boyfriend's sweaters. I loved to wear them on days we weren't together. And I loved to bury my nose in the soft fabric and immerse myself in his scent. Memories of making out or making love would come rushing back to me with all of the attendant desire and arousal. The sensation was so powerful my knees would practically buckle. I could practically *taste* him. And I could hardly wait for my next chance to get my arms around him.

Little did I know at the time, but I was learning a powerful lesson involving stimulus and response—a lesson I want to use to help you recover your most sexy, hot, responsive self. I'm sure you have heard the expression "I want it so bad I can *taste* it" many times. In this chapter I am going to help you taste it so bad you will *want* it. You *need* to stop and think about it more often. And we're going to start right here.

LIVING LIFE IN "SENSE SURROUND"

I know a man whose most powerful sensual memories come from the times when, as a young man, he would go for his monthly haircut. Before each haircut would begin, a beautiful young woman would sensuously shampoo his hair in steaming-hot water and apricot-scented shampoo. He would absolutely lose his mind every time as he watched this beautiful woman so close to him and so focused on him, with her beautiful breasts just inches from touching him. Being way too young to ask the woman out on a date, this was heaven, hell, and everything in between. And it is something he has never forgotten. But the most interesting part of the story for me is that to this day—more than fifteen years later—this man keeps a bottle of apricot-scented shampoo in his shower. Why? Because he can get an erection just by bringing the scent to his nose.

This man lives his life in what I call "sense surround." He isn't afraid to surround himself with the scents that trigger his most erotic memories. And it keeps him feeling sexually connected and sexually charged. Which is exactly how I want you to feel. And that leads me to our first exercise.

"Tasting" Exercise #1

Open your journal to a fresh page. At the top of the page, write:

MY SENSUAL SMELLS ARE:

Now think for a few moments. What are some of the smells that turn you on? It doesn't matter if they are innately erotic, or if you associate them with something erotic. Take at least ten or fifteen minutes to complete this list. Think of every smell that arouses you, soothes you, excites you, or ignites you—roses, jasmine, chocolate, wine, your partner's cologne, your partner's natural body scent, the scent of your partner's penis when you bring it close to your face, the smell of his semen, your own scent on your partner's fingers . . . Don't be afraid of being completely outrageous. I know women who are turned on by the smell of movie theaters because it reminds them of their early sexual escapades. I know women who are turned on by the smell of a new car (perhaps for the same reason!). I even know a few women who are turned on by the smell of gasoline—until they see the price, that is! Are you getting the idea?

"Tasting" Exercise #2

Look at the list you have just completed for "Tasting" Exercise #1. I want you to spend the next fifteen minutes writing about any erotic associations you have just stirred in creating this list. If you remembered a sexually charged moment in your life, write about it. If you're just feeling sexy and tingly, write about it. Immerse yourself in the memories and sensations. Let yourself feel the connection.

NOW INDULGE YOURSELF

How could you live more of your life in "sense surround"? Think about this right now. Look again at the list you have just completed. How could you bring these scents closer to home to eroticize your senses on a regular basis? Is there a cologne you should be keeping by your bedside or dabbing on your pillow? Is there a special fragrance *you* should have in your shower? Should you be holding on to one of your partner's T-shirts? What about bringing home fresh flowers more often, or buying freshly baked loaves of bread? How could you indulge yourself and sexualize your everyday surroundings simply by introducing your special scents? It's time for you to start.

FEEDING THE FLAMES

Food, glorious food. Food, fabulous food. Food, sensual food. If I had written the song, those would have been the lyrics. You may not stop to think about it that often, but the scents, textures, and tastes of food play a big part in creating a sexual mood and context. Let me prove it to you with a simple demonstration. Look at the following two lists:

1. lobster with butter sauce, veal *cordon bleu*, spinach soufflé, pears drizzled with caramel, strawberries and champagne, chocolate mousse

2. fried liver, carrots, cottage cheese, meat loaf, baked potato, burgers, fries, ice water

Which group of foods sounds sexier to you? I know everyone has different tastes, but I *really* hope you said the first group!

Don't get me wrong; I like meat loaf and gravy as much as the next woman, it's just that it doesn't go down on my list of erotic foods. I'm not a nutritionist, so you may not want to quote me on this, but as far as I'm concerned there are only two food groups: food that makes you think about sex, and food that doesn't. And I don't want a balanced diet! When I want to feel more sensual, I surround myself with sensual triggers, and that includes what I eat! To help make the perfect sexual connection you need to create your own sensual surroundings; you need to remodel your environment so that it serves as a constant source of sensual/sexual stimulation for you. And since we all spend so much time in front of our refrigerators, food is the perfect place to begin that remodeling.

This is not a chapter about dieting unless you want to think of it as a "diet for a big, sexy planet." This is a chapter about the erotic powers of taste, texture, and scent, and how to harness these powers and put them to work.

WHEN FOOD IS SEX, THAT'S A GOOD THING

When it comes to being turned on by food, everyone has their favorites. What is on *your* erotic menu? What kinds of foods make you think about sex? Mangoes and papayas? Chocolate-dipped bananas? A bathtub full of baked beans? Whether it's the appearance, the texture, the smell, the taste, or the memories that they trigger, I want to know what foods help you connect to your erotic core. There are, of course, many popular favorites— champagne and caviar, for example, or chocolate ice cream—but I want to know *your* favorites, even if they are things like fried eel or liverwurst spread. And I want you to know them, too, to reconnect to your most powerful associations. And that is what this next exercise is all about.

"Tasting" Exercise #3

Open your journal to a fresh page, get a pen, and start three new lists. At the top of the first list, write:

MY SENSUAL FOODS ARE:

(If it turns you on—no matter what it is—it belongs on the list. It can be a simple food such as vanilla ice cream, or a complex food such as lobster ravioli in a curry cream sauce with a touch of parsley.)

Turn to the next page and write:

MY SENSUAL TASTES ARE:

(What's the difference between tastes and foods? I have a cousin who hates bananas, but loves anything banana flavored. You might also love the taste of cinnamon or vanilla, but I wouldn't call them foods. So go ahead and list all of the **tastes** that turn you on.)

Turn to a third page and write:

MY SENSUAL BEVERAGES ARE:

(This is not supposed to be a list of all of your favorite alcoholic beverages, but a list of beverages whose consistencies, textures, and tastes are particularly sensuous to you. Yes, I love champagne, for example, but when I'm in the mood, a glass of warm milk can be just as sensual.)

Now take at least fifteen minutes to fill in your lists. Try to be comprehensive, even if it means going to the refrigerator right now, or thumbing through your recipe files to refresh your erotic memory.

A TASTE FOR ADVENTURE

Were you aware of all of the various foods and beverages, and the many tastes and smells, that have the capacity to trigger a sensual response in you? Some of the foods on your list may be unhealthy to consume on a regular basis, and I am not encouraging you to give up eating healthy foods and start eating three erotic meals a day. But you now have an arsenal of foods, tastes, and smells that can be used like fuses to help ignite the powder keg that contains your sexual power.

Are you ready to learn how to have some real fun with your food? If you were ever told to "stop playing with your food" as a child, here is your chance to go completely wild.

If you have ever seen the film *9 1/2 Weeks* starring Kim Basinger and Mickey Rourke, you probably have a sneaking suspicion about what is coming next. Talk about having fun with food! Whether you have seen this film a dozen times, or have never seen it, I want you to go to your local video store this afternoon and rent it before reading any farther. The scene you must see before we continue our exercises involves Kim Basinger sitting by an open refrigerator stocked with various food items. The plot of the film may or may not appeal to you, so if you prefer to fast-forward to this one scene and skip the rest of the movie, that's fine with me—I'm a sex therapist, not a film critic!

MAGICALLY DELICIOUS

After you have watched the film, you are ready to review the three lists you compiled in the "Tasting" Exercise #3. What I want you to do now is put a check mark next to all of the items that have a *texture* that is sensual to you—foods that feel good to the *touch*. Limit yourself to single-ingredient items (no baked alaska or bouillabaisse) to keep things simple for now (you'll soon see why!). Some examples would be:

whipped cream
chocolate sauce
milk/chocolate milk
pudding
honey
oatmeal
soft fruits like peaches and strawberries

How many of these items do you have in your house right now? If you have only one or two, or if you don't have any at all (no wonder you're feeling sensually starved!), it's time to make a quick trip to the supermarket. Otherwise, assemble your favorites now and let them come to room temperature. **If any of your items are in glass containers, transfer them into something unbreakable.**

Are you still asking yourself, "Where is this heading?" You don't need to keep guessing. It's heading to the shower where the following exercise will combine elements of touch with elements of taste for a truly sensational experience.

"Tasting" Exercise #4

I call this exercise "the exotic shower." Begin by taking a quick, warm shower. Next, turn the water off and sit in the empty tub. Make sure all of your foods are within reach. Have a bath towel handy, and have some paper towels handy also.

*Start with your **favorite** food. First, take a taste of it. Let it linger in your mouth before you swallow it. Now play with it. Scoop it up, or pour it out, but get it alllll over yourself. **Bathe** in it. Rub it all over your body. Go slowly. And KEEP BREATHING.*

Now, one by one, play with the rest of your sensuous foods. Mash the fruits against yourself. Stick your fingers in your mouth. Pour milk over your head; pour it down cracks and crevices. Drip honey on your breasts. Use the foods as objects and lubricants to give yourself a loving touch.

Go systematically down the line and sample all of your sensuous foods in this way. Take your time, going extra slowly. When you have finished, use the paper towels to scoop up anything that may clog your drain. Turn on the faucet and let the water wash away any slippery elements before you stand up. Wash and dry yourself.

Take a few moments now to reflect on this exercise in your journal. What feelings, fantasies, or memories came up for you? What foods and/or liquids were most pleasurable? When will you do this exercise again? How could you make it even more erotic? Could you imagine "sharing your food" with your partner?

Discovering the extraordinary that resides in the ordinary is one of the things that sexual connection, and developing your extra-sensual perception, are all about. Are you feeling sexier? Are you feeling more alive? Are you amazed by how simple exercises can produce such fabulous results? That's what it means to feel truly connected.

MORE FOOD FOR THOUGHT

I have a client, Joli, whose most powerfully erotic memory in life involves food. Joli was raised in a very strict religious household. As a young adult she was involved with the church choir. The group decided to hold a bake sale to raise funds for an out-of-town singing engagement.

Joli and two other choir members, another young woman and a young man whom she had always found attractive, volunteered to make hand-dipped chocolate-covered strawberries for the sale. On the day the dipping was going to take place, the other young woman become ill and left, so the job fell to Joli and the young man.

Not long into the project, the first strawberry was ready to be dipped. The boy did the honors, and then held the fruit to Joli's lips. As she sank her teeth into the berry, he moved his hand ever so slightly in a circular motion, so that the still warm chocolate clinging to the berry smeared sensuously onto her lips. Although slightly embarrassed, she reports that licking the chocolate off her lips while he watched created the most profoundly arousing sensation she had ever experienced up to that point in her life.

Next, it was his turn to taste. She dipped a berry for him, then held it to his lips. When he took a bite, she smeared the chocolate on his lips, as he had done with her. Her heart raced as she watched him begin to lick the chocolate from his mouth. He took another strawberry, dipped it, and then used the tip of it to apply chocolate directly to Joli's lips. Without warning, he leaned in and kissed her. The combination of the urgent kiss and the sweet, warm chocolate was the first time my client had ever experienced sexual passion. I am sure it is not hard for you to understand why this woman can recall those feelings any time she even *thinks* of chocolate-covered strawberries.

You may not have an erotic memory involving food that is as clear-cut as the one described above, but I'll bet if you think about it, you will be able to recall many foods that played a part, either large or small, in some of your most memorable sexual encounters.

"Tasting" Exercise #5

Open your journal to a fresh page. Think back now and compose a list of food and drink that you can recall as being a part of a sensual, erotic, or sexual experience you once had. Were you roasting marshmallows around a campfire the first time you kissed? Or what about the cheese fondue you shared right before making love on the living room floor when you were newlyweds? Were you ever fed shrimp cocktail while being "fingered" under the table in a fancy restaurant?

Keep going in this vein and try to excavate as many memories involving food and sexual excitement as you possibly can.

"Tasting" Exercise #6

I like to think of this exercise as "The Lust Supper." Pick an evening you can devote to a long dinner. On this evening you are going to create a "lust" supper for yourself by assembling a banquet of foods that were on hand during some of the hottest moments in your sexual history. From your first sip of an aperitif to the last morsel of cake, everything should have an erotic attachment. If you are having trouble remembering many foods in this context, you can supplement your meal with foods from the "sensual foods list" you compiled earlier.

This is the first exercise in the book in which you can involve your partner. After all, he's got to eat, too! HOWEVER, keep the motivation behind the meal to yourself. If the food is from a memory that involves him, you may simply want to remind him of the event when you serve it. You obviously would not want to risk hurting your partner's feelings by relating a sexual story that did **not** involve him. Let whatever happens happen, and try not to hold any expectations as to what **should** happen between you.

Your goal is to try to **connect with the sexual feelings** you associate with each particular taste. If any shared memories or your state of arousal should happen to lead to intimacy between you and your partner, great! Enjoy it! But remember, your focus is still on you at this point, and there is **no pressure** on either of you to respond or perform in any particular way.

While you are eating try to:

1. *Recall the time of day, the temperature, the lighting, and the other physical details involved in each sensual memory.*
2. *Vividly replay the scene in your mind's eye.*
3. *Allow yourself to fully experience the textures and tastes of everything you are eating and drinking.*
4. *Immerse yourself in the sensual/sexual feelings that accompany each scene you are recalling.*
5. *Flex your PC muscle periodically to help stimulate your erotic response and keep you focused.*

(If you have no erotic food memories, try to create some during this exercise by thinking of a particularly hot, sexy experience you had and, with your imagination, inserting sensuous food into the scene as a prelude to the event or as a part of the event.)

Are you starting to see how the sexual potential already lives inside you and how, with just a little bit of effort and imagination, you can stoke the fire until the connection is red-hot? The quality of our experiences adds up to the quality of our lives. The more we are capable of squeezing each juicy drop out of *every* experience we have had, do have, and will have, the more fully we will have lived. In this chapter we made quite a few glasses of sensual juice—figuratively, and perhaps even literally. In the next chapter we open the floodgates.

5

Playing

*i*n the previous chapters you reestab-
lished a physical and erotic connection
with your body. You became intimate
with its shape, textures, and strength,
and you rediscovered (or perhaps discovered for the very first time) the way
that you can be aroused with specific
touches, tastes, and smells.

The work that you have already done in this
short period of time will provide the solid foundation upon which you can now build. And,
according to my blueprints, it's time for the rec
room to go in! That means it's time to bring in
the toys.

TOYS, TOYS, TOYS

When we were children, one of the fastest ways
of gaining access to our imaginations and
enhancing our sense of play was through the
introduction of a toy. We are no longer children,

but toys still have the power to delight and
amuse us, focus and teach us, free and enlighten
us. In fact, one of the best ways to lighten up,
brighten up, and bring a whole new level of
excitement to your sex life is by becoming familiar and learning to play with . . . sexual toys.

If you wanted to paint, the very first thing you
would do would be to surround yourself with art
supplies and inspiration. You would buy a wide
variety of paints, pastels, and crayons. You'd buy
a wide variety of brushes and palette knives.
You'd buy different papers and different can-
vases. Everything you could do to encourage
and tease out your creativity would become a
part of your surroundings. Well, it isn't all that
different when it comes to teasing out your sexual energy and aliveness.

To step into your sexual power and gain access
to your wildest sexual self, you need to immerse
yourself in erotic surroundings by filling your
world with sex toys and assorted sexual paraphernalia. What *kind* of toys and paraphernalia
am I talking about? A dildo, for example. That's
right, an artificial phallus. (Maybe, to help break
the ice, you need to say the word "dildo" out
loud a few times before we continue.) You need
at least one dildo, and it would better if you had
several. You also need: a vibrator, a smattering of
flavored lubricants, a few XXX videos, some

nasty lingerie, a pair of sexy high heels, and anything else you can think of that will bring you
closer to your erotic essence and reveal your sexual core. And you need to have a toy chest—a
box or drawer safe from prying eyes where you
can keep your private "stash" when you aren't in
the mood to play.

A BLUE SHOPPING SPREE

If the aspiring artist visits an art-supply store to
stock up on the essentials, your interests will
take you to one of the many nonthreatening and
professional adult "toy stores" that can be found
today in most cities across the country.

If you have never visited a sex store before,
you may feel some apprehension at the thought
of doing so. But here's my professional advice:
Do it anyway. I will be very surprised if the experience doesn't somehow arouse and embolden
you, or at least put an "I've-got-a-secret" smile
on your face! If you need to, ask a friend to go
with you for support. Turn it into a ladies' night
out if you have to. But the experience will be
well worth the effort.

If you absolutely, positively cannot handle
such a public forum for an X-rated adventure,
shopping by catalog or via the Internet is the
next best thing, and it's what I recommend for

you. I also recommend these two shop-at-home alternatives if there isn't an appropriate, professionally run store in your area. **Please don't go visiting scary stores in marginal neighborhoods.** Refer to the Appendix at the back of this book for a list of professionally run, discreet mail-order companies and on-line services that can help you shop at home for everything you need.

MAKING A LIST, CHECKING IT TWICE

Every shopping spree goes more smoothly when there is a master plan, and your shopping spree is no different. Making a list before you venture into the store will: one, act as a touchstone to keep you grounded and focused should you find yourself overwhelmed by the plethora of merchandise on display; and two, guarantee that you won't just scurry in and scurry out without having a good, full look at the amazing variety of toys, games, clothing, and equipment available for your pleasure. Who knows, you may even make an impulse buy!

Here are some items for your list:

1. *At least one penis-shaped dildo.*
    You will probably see dildos that vary
    greatly in size, texture, and shape. A

good way to break the ice is to find a phallus that reminds you most of your man's. It should be shaped to look like a real penis (not smooth or missile-like), and be crafted from soft rubber or a jellylike substance. If it also vibrates, so much the better. If your budget allows, splurge on a few different sizes. Get a dildo designed to stimulate your G-spot (it will have a curved neck), or one with "ribs" or "ticklers."

2. *A vibrator.*
   Specifically, a handheld clitoral stimulator. This type of vibrator is not penis shaped and is designed for external use only. Often it has a variety of massaging heads that can be attached, but most often it comes with a short, detachable tip with a ball-like end. (These types of vibrators are often available in larger drugstores as well.)

3. *Lubricant.*
   You will definitely need a water-based, lubricating gel for use with your dildo. No need to limit yourself to just KY jelly anymore; pick a few of your favorite flavors and/or scents.

4. *Sexy lingerie.*

   This purchase may require a separate stop at a special lingerie store if the sex shop does-n't carry lingerie. Fight the urge to play it safe. Instead, choose something that feels dangerous to you; something that is absolutely, undeniably, and categorically designed for sex. Think XXX here, not romance novels. The more outrageous the better.

5. *One or two erotic videos.*

   You've had the thoughts—now see the movie! You might prefer films directed by women, but I couldn't know your tastes. The descriptions on the boxes will help you choose.

6. *"Try-it-once" items.*

   If it's something you'd like to try just one time—just out of curiosity, if nothing more—put it on the list. Who knows, it could be just the beginning of something new and beautiful.

Now shop till you drop!

NOTICE YOUR POST-SHOPPING GLOW

On your way home from your very grown-up shopping spree, take note of what you are think-

ing about. Are you thinking about your work?
Are you thinking about your weight? Are you
thinking about who to vote for in the next elec-
tion? I doubt it.

My guess is, you're thinking about sex. You're
thinking about that bundle of goodies in the
trunk and how using it is going to make you feel.

Are you feeling sexy? Are you feeling proud?
Are you feeling your temperature rise? You
should be. By purchasing these items, you have
made a declaration to your psyche that you are a
very sexual being. No more hiding from yourself. You have made a conscious decision to put
the "life" back into your sex life. And, as a result,
you are *instantly* feeling the connection. I'll bet it
feels great!

TIME TO PLAY

Do you remember recess? Do you remember
how your anticipation would grow so that when
the bell finally rang you would catapult out of
your seat and hit the playground running? You
would play with reckless abandon, and it was
delicious.

Safe at home now with all your new toys, a
whole different kind of anticipation is building
up inside you. You are ready to play! Well, if I
am the teacher and you are the student, then I

get to say when it is time for recess . . . and it's time for recess! It's time to immerse yourself in your many purchases. It's time to play with reckless abandon. You have the anticipation, you have the desire, and you have all the necessary equipment. There is only one thing left to find: You need the right *place* to play.

FINDING YOUR PRIVATE PLAYGROUND

Playing with your grown-up toys is a very private affair. During your introduction to this adventure, you need to be alone, you need to feel safe, and you need to be free of distractions and interruptions. Perhaps your bedroom is the place to begin the next exercise. But then again, perhaps it isn't. Too much dirty laundry, too many ringing telephones, too many bills on the desk . . . this may not be conducive to play. If your bedroom feels less than ideal for your first encounter with your toys, may I suggest a more exciting alternative: your own private hotel or motel room.

Renting a hotel or motel room for the afternoon, or even staying for an evening (if your lifestyle and commitments allow for that), is the perfect way to turbocharge the next exercise. It may sound a little extravagant, but if there was ever a time to splurge on yourself, trust me when I tell you that this *is* the time. It's not that your bedroom at home is necessarily a bad place. But nothing frees you more than getting away from your usual environment—even if it's for just a few hours.

We want to coax that devilish side of you to come out and play hard. The more you get away from familiar surroundings, the more you open up the possibility for something, and *someone*, new to emerge. Hotels and motels have powerful associations with illicit affairs and "naughty" sex. So what better place to continue your "illicit affair"—the one you are having with *yourself*— than in a place where things feel very private and you feel a little bit pampered.

CHECK-IN TIME IS NOW

If you decide to go to a hotel or motel room for this next exercise, be sure to pack and bring with you:

1. your dildo, vibrator, and lubricants
2. your sexy lingerie
3. a pair of sexy high-heeled shoes
4. bath oil
5. a radio or portable CD player with headphones
6. extra batteries if any of your toys are battery operated

7. candles
8. your videos (your room may have a VCR)
9. your sex journal

If for some reason you cannot rent a hotel/motel room, don't struggle with your decision. If you can be home *alone* for a few hours, that's the next best thing. But do everything you can to approximate the experience of being out of the house. For example, turn off the ringer on your telephone so it won't disturb you. If you're going to leave your answering machine on, turn the volume down. And mentally hang a DO NOT DISTURB sign.

A RENDEZVOUS FOR ONE

Have you checked into your hotel/motel room? Congrats! Your heart is probably beating faster already. If your hotel has room service, perhaps you would like to order a bite to eat first. (If you're at home, have food delivered.) I recommend something indulgent and slightly decadent, such as a giant shrimp cocktail or a big hot-fudge sundae. Refer back to your lists from the previous chapter for more ideas. Remember that the whole thrust (pun intended!) of this exercise is to have fun and do what feels good to you.

Before continuing, be sure to double-lock (or chain) all doors and draw all the curtains closed—you don't need any unwelcome surprises or nosy neighbors. Even if you are at home, you need to make sure no one (spouse, children, etc.) can make a sudden appearance.

After your meal, draw a warm bath for yourself. Fill the tub with fragrant oils or bubble bath. Fully undress, if you have not done so already. Lower yourself into the water and take several cleansing sensual breaths. When you are feeling relaxed, begin a slow, sensuous, full-body loving touch. Take as much time as you need. When you are finished, step out of the bath, and towel off. It's time for the exercises.

"Playing" Exercise #1

Double-check that the doors are securely locked/chained and the curtains are all closed. Lower the lights, light a few candles, and turn on some soft, sexy music. Slip into your naughty lingerie and sexy pumps so you are feeling "dressed to thrill." Now look at yourself in a mirror. How does wearing such a blatantly sexual outfit make you feel? Does it make you move differently? Is it turning you on?

Strike as many sexy and provocative poses as you can think of. Feel yourself up while you say nasty things to yourself. Tell yourself how hot you look. There's nobody there but you, so you can really let yourself go.

*Be the nastiest **you** you can possibly be.*

"Playing" Exercise #2

Place your toys where you can reach them easily from the bed. If any of your equipment is electric, plug it in. If you have a VCR in the room, you may want to start playing one of your tapes. Now relax, get comfortable, and take several deep, cleansing breaths.

What I want you to do now is grab your dildo and pretend it's your lover's penis. Feel every ripple and ridge. Stare at it. Kiss it. Give it a long, languorous lick. Suck it, if you like. Now apply a generous amount of lubricant to the phallus. It is very important that the dildo remain well lubricated at all times for the rest of this exercise. I cannot overemphasize what a difference it will make in your enjoyment of the experience.

Slowly insert the head of the dildo into your vagina. Allow yourself time to get used to the new sensations. Slowly add an inch of the dildo at a time. When you have fitted as much of it into your vagina as you can comfortably hold, remove your hand and let the dildo rest inside you for a moment. Is your PC muscle pulsing? Now hold the dildo in place and squeeze it with your PC muscle several times. Do you feel your pump getting primed?

When you are ready, begin a slow and easy thrust. Make sure to keep the dildo extremely well lubricated. As you are ready, slowly increase the speed of your thrusting. You may find the hard ridge of the head is especially stimulating to your G-spot as you withdraw. If you feel your arousal level building to orgasm, go ahead and ride the wave. If you are not building to orgasm with the dildo, please don't *worry about it. Although having an orgasm is fabulous, your main goal is simply to make yourself feel good.*

If you *have* climaxed using the dildo, you may want to give yourself some time to recover before embarking on this next exercise.

"Playing" Exercise #3

Continuing from "Playing" Exercise #2, it is time now to turn on your vibrator. If the vibrator has more than one speed, start with the lowest, or slowest, speed. It is not necessary to apply lubricant to the vibrator, but it is fine if some lubricant remains on your genitals or if you would like to apply some to yourself.

To get a feel for the strength of your vibrator, start by applying the tip to the palm of your hand. Move the tip in slow circles using varying degrees of pressure. When you feel comfortable, move down to your genitals.

Lightly touch the hood of your clitoris with the vibrating tip. If this is the first time you have ever used a vibrator, the feeling may be extremely intense for you; you may need to disengage often between touches. If it doesn't feel too intense, try varying the amount of pressure you apply, your movements, and the speed.

Be gentle with yourself. Everything you are feeling should be pleasurable to you. If you feel any discomfort, you are probably using too much pressure. Keep your touch light until your vibrator becomes more familiar to you. Go at your own speed.

If you are like a lot of women, you may come to orgasm very quickly using the vibrator; in fact, you may have one of the most explosive orgasms you have ever experienced. Relax and enjoy it. You deserve to have that kind of pleasure. If you didn't, you wouldn't have been born with the equipment!

If you did not climax with your vibrator, that is perfectly okay. There is no contest or race to be won here. The important thing is that you are doing what is pleasurable to you. If you did bring yourself to orgasm with the vibrator, you may want to catch your breath before proceeding to the next exercise.

"Playing" Exercise #4

*You are going to need your dildo **and** your vibrator for this exercise. ($1 + 1 = $ WOW!) Slather lubricant onto your dildo. Slowly insert it into your vagina. Begin a slow thrusting motion as you did in "Playing" Exercise #1 and let your arousal build. When you're ready, switch on the vibrator with your other hand. Bring the vibrator head to your clitoral hood as you did in the previous exercise. Feel your vagina clamp down around the dildo. This is your PC muscle at work. Continue thrusting with the dildo as you stimulate your clitoris with the vibrator. Feel the intensity of your arousal continue to build. Play with your level of arousal: Withdraw the vibrator periodically, or stop your thrusting to feel the intensity of your pleasure peak and drop* *off. Use your dildo and vibrator to work your body up and down till you're absolutely spent. What a combo!*

Although orgasm has not been the goal, I wouldn't be surprised if you had at least one orgasm from this last exercise, if not several. All the stimulation may even have triggered a "gusher." A gusher is an extremely pleasurable type of orgasm that is marked by an ejaculation of clear, thin fluid. This phenomenon is often triggered by intense stimulation of the G-spot. (The G-spot is located on the top wall of your vagina, about two thirds of the way up, and it is extremely sensitive.) For some women, the ejaculation is forceful and literally shoots out of them. Others just notice a considerable amount of the clear fluid running down their legs. In either case, a gusher is cause for celebration, as it is an indication that you have been deeply and profoundly stimulated.

COMING BACK DOWN TO EARTH

I hope this chapter has helped to open up your mind, your eyes, your heart, and your body to the great depths of sexual pleasure and satisfaction that you are capable of receiving and experiencing. You just had great sex! And you did it all by yourself. Just imagine what it will be like

when you bring this same newfound energy, creativity, and freedom into lovemaking with your
partner! Imagine the power of your connection!
I'm betting that neither of you will ever be the
same; and that's the whole point, isn't it? But it's
still early in the journey, and time to continue to
Level II . . .

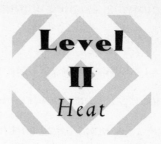

Level II
Heat

In Level I of this book, you saw how it is possible to stimulate and energize sexual feeling through physical touch, taste, and movement, and how to establish a connection with your erotic core. In Level II your focus will travel up your body from the purely physical (relating to the groin) to the emotional and the mental (relating to the heart and the mind).

We have all heard the saying at one time or another that 90 percent of sex takes place "between the ears." After having completed Level I, I will understand if you want to adjust that percentage a bit! But it is the truth of the matter that, although your body provides the way that you have sex, your thoughts and emotions provide the will to have sex. And without the **will**, there is no way you will have *satisfying, exciting, nurturing, creative sex with your partner.*

In Level I you got your body primed for an extraor-dinary, lasting sexual connection. In Level II you will get your mind and heart to follow.

6

Wanting

*t*his is a chapter about sexual desire—the luscious feeling of "wanting" sex. And our goal here is to amplify the budding feelings of desire that have been emerging from your commitment to making an unforgettable sexual connection. But what exactly *is* sexual desire? Is it something chemical? Is it something psychological? Is it something spiritual? Is it, as so many people believe, the same as sexual *drive*? And does it really matter as long as you're having sex?

As a sex therapist and author it is my purpose and my joy to enlighten my clients and readers through playful, pleasurable, and, hopefully, meaningful exercises that require your active participation. But occasionally the Ph.D. in me climbs up to the lectern and won't budge until it has had its say. The subject of "drive versus desire" definitely brings out that side of me.

I passionately believe that simply understanding the difference between sexual desire and sexual drive, and how differently they operate within you, can prove to be a turning point in the sex life of many women, and a cornerstone in your sexual connection. Too many of us get confused by the fluctuations in our sexual appetites and imaginations and reach many of the wrong conclusions. We blame chemistry for problems shaped by our mind-sets; we blame our mind-sets for problems shaped by changes in our chemistry. And the end result is frustration and lack of fulfillment. Sexual desire and sexual drive are *not* the same thing. They are not interchangeable. They are not even similar. And my goal in this chapter is to make the difference clear.

But I'm going to stop the lecture here. Instead of offering textbook definitions of "desire" and "drive," and loading you up with pages of notes, I want to try a slightly different approach. I would like to offer first a memorable story—a story that paints a vivid picture of that thing called desire, and a very different picture of that thing we call drive. These two pictures, each worth far more than a thousand words, are snapshots I would like you to always have in your mind's eye. They will help you form your own definitions, and a much more comprehensive personal understanding as well.

◈

Two women friends, Sally and Joan, are out together on a blind double date. They meet the men, whom we will call Robert and Hank, at a local restaurant. They all have a drink at the bar and say their hellos before moving to a table where they proceed to order dinner.

Although neither of these men is really her "type," Sally initially finds Hank the better looking of the two. Yet over the course of the evening, Sally is amazed to find herself absolutely captivated by *Robert*. He's smart, interesting, funny, considerate, and quietly sexy. She feels an electric current when their eyes meet and they are talking as if they have known each other forever. The attentive and appreciative way he looks at her makes her feel womanly and powerful; the extra two pounds she discovered during her morning weigh-in seem immaterial in the face of the strong, positive feelings she is currently enjoying. As they continue to talk and laugh, Sally starts to fantasize about kissing him, touching him, him touching her. . . . She is imagining herself on future dates with him; she wants to get to know him better. She can feel excitement and heat stirring in her belly. She *wants* him.

So what about Joan? Joan happened to wake *up* that morning wanting sex. The ache is so strong that on the way up to her office in an elevator full of people she forgot herself and complained to a coworker, "I'm *so* horny I could die!" Even a couple of men who she *knows* find her attractive couldn't wait to get off the elevator and away from the undiscriminating hunger of Joan's blind need.

The minute Joan lays eyes on their dates that evening she is relieved to see that either of them could qualify as a viable candidate. They seem to have all their fingers and toes and she quickly learns that they are capable of performing simple tasks ("Hand me a napkin? Thank you.").

At dinner it soon becomes apparent that her friend Sally is falling for . . . what's his name again? Anyway, the one with the sexy bald spot. What*ever*! The other one, this blond guy here, will do *just fine*! She can see his mouth moving, but Joan isn't hearing much of his conversation. She's trying to guess his penis size and praying she remembered to put a few condoms in her purse. She sure hopes that third glass of wine doesn't interfere with his getting an erection! Joan isn't thinking about the past, and she couldn't care less about the future. She isn't interested in learning what Hank's hobbies are, his likes or dislikes, or whether he's seen any good movies lately. She cares about one thing and one thing only: her need to get laid, and how quickly she and this guy can get out of here so that he can be of service to her.

One woman consumed by her desire, another woman consumed by her drive. Is it clear to you which is which? Please understand that I am not making value judgments on what the two women in this story are experiencing. Both desire and drive are necessary to make and sustain sexual connection. And as you can see, both desire and drive contribute to a woman's hunger for sexual intimacy. But that is pretty much where the similarities end.

It is Joan who is demonstrating evidence of a sex *drive* in high gear. And, believe it or not, Joan's sex drive is fueled primarily by testosterone, the same hormone responsible for a man's sex drive. The female sex drive is a physiological response that evolves fluidly in keeping with the hormonal changes in her life. These changes are affected by major events such as surgery, pregnancy, childbirth, and menopause. Birth control pills and other synthetic substances also affect sex drive because of the way they artificially regulate the flow of hormones. But it is hormones that are the key to drive—Joan's drive, and your drive.

(Note: If you are concerned that you have lost your sex drive, and your life conditions haven't changed significantly—you remain in love with your partner, you are not unduly stressed, you have not started any hormonal medications— there may be a biological cause for this that merits investigation. I recommend that you consult an endocrinologist.)

So what about *desire*?

Sally is experiencing all of the exquisite symptoms of sexual desire. But it is not hormones that are fueling her fire right now. It is important for you to understand that desire is nourished primarily by mind-set—Sally's mind-set, and *your* mind-set. Desire results from a complex interplay of factors, including self-esteem and self-acceptance, the level of permission we give ourselves to express our sexuality, contextual elements as minute and idiosyncratic to each woman as stress level, physical settings, and temperature, and, as this story clearly illustrates, our feelings toward our partner—our feelings overall, and our feelings in the moment. Desire, then, more than anything, is really about feelings; feelings you have the power to change.

YOU'RE DE DAME, HE'S DE SIRE

A pop quiz: In a minute's time, write down every positive attribute you can think of belonging to your partner. Don't labor over your responses; there are no wrong or right answers. Just jot down as many qualities describing him as you can think of. You've got one minute. Ready? Set? Go!

I'm sure you wrote down many interesting things. Maybe aspects of his personality you have begun to take for granted or don't give him enough credit for. It is important to acknowledge your partner's good qualities whenever you can. Start thanking him whenever you are sincerely grateful for anything he has done, from putting the toilet seat down to giving you an orgasm.

But here is my question: How many of you wrote the word "man" on your list describing your mate? That's a good thing, remember? Personally, I don't believe that familiarity breeds contempt as much as it breeds numbness and blindness. We get so wrapped up in thinking of our partner in terms of his role as a husband or boyfriend or father or provider or whatever it is he does for a living that we lose sight of one very basic, fundamental, and *crucial* aspect of his makeup: He's a *man*, honey! You've got yourself a man! Remember when you didn't have one? Remember how badly you wanted one? Well, there he is. So write it on your list this very minute!

It is necessary to reclaim your perception of your partner as *a man* in order to begin awakening the desire that slumbers within you. Forget that he's your husband, or your children's father, or that you've known him for the past fifteen years. It's time to get amnesia. Don't even think of him as *your* man. He's a man who's got something that you want—something that you *need*. And in the next exercise I'm going to show you one way to use that simple fact to fill you with desire.

BUILDING DESIRE

To prepare for this exercise, gather together the items you use for your loving touch, including massage oil, genital lubricant, and a towel. You will also be using a blindfold, so locate a scarf or sleep mask.

Now open your partner's underwear drawer. Does he have a sexy pair of briefs that you love—something silky, slinky, or just cut in a sexy way? Boxers are okay too if that's your thing. They can be brand new, or they can be ones you've seen him in a hundred times; the only criterion for them is that they turn *you* on. If your partner doesn't live with you, ask him to bring an extra pair with him the next time he visits. You don't need to give him a long explanation; let his own imagination fill him with desire, too.

(Please note: If you're not quite ready to go this far out on a limb, start with a T-shirt right now, and work your way "down" from there over the course of time.)

Now select a favorite cologne or aftershave of his and spray or dab a little bit onto his shorts. Take everything you have assembled and get into bed to prepare for a very special loving touch. Put on your blindfold, apply your massage oil, and begin the exercise.

"Wanting" Exercise #1

Start with a series of slow, deep, cleansing breaths. Focus your attention on the air going in through your nose and out through your mouth. Be present in your body. Begin touching yourself lightly with your fingertips. Whatever your speed is, cut it in half. Slow and sensuous is the name of the game. Continue your loving touch and let your arousal start to build.

*Now bring your lover's undergarment to your face. Inhale his scent deeply. Feel the soft material against your skin. Picture your partner's hard penis straining against the thin fabric. Wherever you touch yourself with his briefs, imagine that his penis is rubbing you, poking you, prodding you. Apply lubricant to your vagina and begin masturbating using your hand. As you continue to masturbate, I want you to have what I call a "**fantasticus interruptus**"—a fantasy with a sudden premature ending. Try something like this:*

The two of you are strangers to each other, alone in an elevator. Suddenly everything goes dark and the elevator comes to a halt. You're panicked, but the stranger takes your hand and tells you that everything is going to be all right. You smell his clean scent as his strong hand caresses the back of your neck. He comes to stand behind you and he presses his erection against your buttocks. His scent grows stronger and it intoxicates you. His hand reaches under your skirt and his fingers slip between the crotch of your panties and your skin. With a beckoning motion, he slowly strokes your clit with his middle finger. You don't know why you're allowing this strange man to do this to you, but you are. In fact, you're soaking wet. He plunges his finger deep inside you. You feel your clit swell and you turn to let your open mouth fall on his. You're frantically working to remove his belt. He has ripped off your blouse, and is simultaneously suckling your breasts and unzipping your skirt. As the skirt slides down your stockinged legs, he falls to his knees, yanks down your panties and buries his head between your thighs. You have never felt anything so divine. You slither to the floor where you feel your mystery lover finally slip his hard penis inside you. You cry out with pleasure as he enters you! You have never been more excited. But suddenly there is movement—and light! The elevator has started again and is moving swiftly down to the lobby floor . . .

CUT! End of fantasy! DO NOT LET YOURSELF GO OVER THE EDGE INTO ORGASM. Leave yourself panting and longing for your lover. Leave yourself *wanting. Do you feel that? That's desire in its purest form. It's excruciating and delicious at the same time, isn't it? Let the unfulfilled desire resonate within you and create a sense of intense longing for your partner. The longing that you feel can act as a bridge, reconnecting you to a sense of sexual urgency in your life and in your relationship. Let it linger!*

I'VE GOT A SEXY SECRET

You know how you feel the day after a night of great sex? You walk around feeling sensual all day long; there's a spring in your step, and maybe you hum a little tune. Images from the night before replay themselves in your mind's eye, bringing a little Mona Lisa smile to your lips at the oddest times: at work, in the check-out line at the grocery store, or stopped at a red light. You might shudder with pleasure or find yourself lubricating just by thinking about what you and your partner did together. Your evening of passion is your sexy secret to draw energy, pleasure, and confidence from all day long. And it keeps you constantly connected to your sense of "wanting."

What if it were possible to switch the order of this fabulous scenario? Instead of starting with lovemaking, what if it were possible to *start* with a sexy secret that kindled your desire and led you *into* a night of passionate sex? I think you know me well enough by now to know that I wouldn't lead you down the garden path without giving you a rose! It *is* possible to come in through the "back door" of this equation and arrive at the same erotic destination.

The day after a night of great sex, you are still enjoying many pleasing *physical* sensations, as well as the mental and emotional lift. You may feel as if your entire vagina is twitching—from the lips to the cervix. Your PC muscle has probably gotten a thorough workout and is still mildly spasming from time to time. This fills you with pleasure, and brings your mind right back to where it belongs, which is on SEX, of course! It's a beautiful loop, is it not? And because it is a loop, you can jump on at *any point* in the sequence; this story does not have to have a beginning, a middle, and an end— it can be endless! This means you don't have to wait for your partner or depend on the elements of chance to get the ball rolling. Instead, you can *start* with the afterglow—start with the sexy secret— and let it work like "abracadabra" all day long on the doors that open to a deep, sexual connection with yourself and the one you want.

I'm going to show you how to jump on this joy ride and summon all of the lingering sensations great sex brings by creating sexy secrets. I am going to point out many roads, all of which lead to

Rome, but only *you* are capable of knowing which road or roads you are most comfortable taking. I am respectful of the fact that one woman's walk on the wild side is another woman's walk in the park, so I will suggest many variations on this same theme. I hope that those among you who tend to be more inhibited will "work up" to the variations that may strike you as being rather exotic. And I also hope that even those of you who consider yourselves adventurous will try the variations that may, at first glance, seem a little tame. But you are in control; make the decisions that are comfortable for you, and set a pace that is comfortable for you.

SEXY SECRET #1: DON'T WEAR UNDERWEAR

Remember the famous interrogation scene in *Basic Instinct* with Sharon Stone? Years later, people are *still* talking about it. Why is it so sexy? Because it is so unexpected. Only *bad* girls don't wear underwear; it feels totally taboo.

Your skirt doesn't have to be as short as Sharon Stone's, but it should definitely be a skirt. You want to be able to feel the air caressing you. Also, when you wear a skirt, every time you walk or cross your legs the weight will put pressure directly on your most sensitive spots; when you wear pants, the material gets in the way.

You don't want to do this on a workday—not yet, anyway. And you don't want to go any place where you feel too vulnerable (on public transportation, for example) or where it would be completely inappropriate. It might be enough to just walk around the house this way for an entire day. Or to try it on an afternoon walk with your partner, or when you go to the movies together. Wherever you try it, I guarantee you that the sensation of being completely exposed underneath your skirt will completely titillate and arouse you. You will find yourself automatically flexing your PC muscle due to the increased stimulation you are experiencing. You will be feeling *very* sexy.

SEXY SECRET #2: SHAVE YOUR PUBIC HAIR

Shaving your pubic hair is another effective way of focusing on your sexual energy. It literally brings your sex out of hiding from behind a "bush" and into the open where it can be seen, admired, felt, and appreciated.

Some women like leaving a tiny patch or "strip" of hair, but it can be even more exciting to shave off *everything*. Even the *act* of shaving off all your pubic hair can feel very erotic. Always use lots of soap or shaving gel, and a brand-new safety razor. If your pubic hair is especially thick or dense, trim it with scissors first. Unlike your legs, you want to shave in the *same direction that the hair grows.*

In the same way that your head would feel very sensitive and exposed if it were shaved, your pubic mound and entire vaginal area will feel nuder than nude with the hair removed. After you have gone pantiless once or twice, try going without underwear after having denuded yourself for an even more erotic experience!

SEXY SECRET #3: SPEND THE DAY WITH YOUR PC MUSCLE

Now that you have discovered and strengthened your PC muscle, spend an entire day checking in and feeling its strength. Start in the shower with a series of flexes. Do another series while you're having your morning coffee. Do a series on your way to work, and another series when you get to work. Do a series at lunch, and another at the gym. Boldly flex every time you're in a roomful of men, or in a crowded elevator—no one will know but you, and it will make you feel sexy and powerful. Rest between "sets"—you don't want to burn yourself out—but keep coming back to it all day along. Flex a few times when your partner walks in the door. Flex a few times when you kiss. Do a series of flexes throughout your dinner and you'll be ready to have your partner for dessert.

SEXY SECRET #4: SPEND THE DAY WITH "HIM"

Sure he's got to go to work, and you probably can't spend the day with the genuine article. But you've got an article of his clothing to keep you company—i.e., the shorts you used in "Desire" Exercise #1, dabbed with his cologne—and that can produce some pretty genuine feelings of desire throughout the day if you put them in your handbag and keep them close to you. Sneak a peak on a regular basis. Feel the texture with your hands, and take in the sexy scent. Think of how they felt to you during the exercise. Think of him.

SEXY SECRET #5: WEAR A STRAP-ON VIBRATOR

Have I lost my mind? No, but you will lose yours if you try this secret on. It may sound a little wacky, or way too far over the edge, but if you can get past that, this will feel like one of the boldest, most purely sexual, *dirty* things you have ever done in your life; in other words, you'll love it!

Either at your local sex shop, or in any of the catalogs I have listed for you in the Appendix of this book, you will find what is commonly referred to as a "butterfly" vibrator. The butterfly is so named because the two- to three-inch vibrating "egg" that lies over your pubic mound and clitoris is connected to two small wings through which the straps are attached. The vibrator is quiet and is powered by two AA batteries. Most allow you to regulate the speed and are specifically designed to be worn under clothing. (But that doesn't mean you should wear it outside your house—not yet, anyway.) Turn it on for a minute or two at first, then turn it on for a little longer. You probably wouldn't want to keep it turned on for a very long time, but you can certainly *wear* it for a long time. *Even if you never turn it on*, just *wearing* the butterfly vibrator under your clothing will be pretty darn exciting.

When you're wearing a strap-on, your body and mind will never let you forget that you are a highly charged sexual being. Give yourself permission to try it at least once; if you don't like it, you never have to do it again. But if you do like it, you have made a discovery that can heighten your level of eroticism and bring you pleasure whenever you want to feel more sexually connected!

MORE SEXY SECRETS

There are many other sexy secrets you can induge in, like wearing a bra that exposes your nipples, wearing crotchless panties and garters, and using *ben wa* balls (small metal balls that you insert into your vagina and hold there) to stimulate your PC muscle into action. What sexy secrets can you think of that would be safe and fun for you to try? Even going braless can feel pretty sexy if it's something you never, ever do. Write down your ideas as they occur to you and try them one by one. Have fun with it!

Isn't it exciting to learn that there is such a simple and immediate way of juicing up your sexiness quotient that is completely in your control and right at your fingertips?

No One Knows What Goes On Behind Your Clothes

Perhaps the greatest hurdle to get over in regard to creating your own sexy secrets is the sensation that everyone you encounter has suddenly developed X-ray vision and knows exactly what's going on under your skirt (or in your handbag). NO ONE WILL KNOW UNLESS YOU DECIDE TO TELL THEM. And you really should resist the temptation to tell anyone, even your best female friend. The incredible power of this exercise lies in its secret nature. Having a sexy secret, and keeping that sexy secret all to yourself, makes it far more luscious and electrifying.

WHY ALL THE SECRETS?

When you serve a nice dinner, it doesn't just appear on the table. You have put a fair amount of work into getting it there. First, you had to visualize it. You have held a picture of the dish you want to create in your mind's eye. Second, you have spent time tending to the various ingredients; you have stirred, basted, tasted, and stirred some more. Why in the world should great sex require any less preparation than a great meal?

Your sexy secret is the main ingredient in a recipe for a night (or afternoon!) of great sex. It is the stirring, the basting, and the marinating that culminates in your diving into the NC-17 casserole that's simmering in your mind's eye.

When you consider how far down on the list of priorities your sexual health and vitality usually are, it should become quite clear to you why semi-drastic measures such as these are necessary to shake loose the cobwebs that bind you to your ordinary ways of thinking and behaving. You don't need to do these things every day, but

you can effect dramatic and permanent change
by making sexy secrets a regular part of your
lovemaking ritual.

THE YOU NOBODY KNOWS

As you move more deeply into forming a lasting
connection with your sexual self, you may feel as
though you are casting off an old shell, much in
the same way that certain animals shed their
skins as they outgrow them. I hope that this is
true for you and that you are enjoying the journey that you have embarked on.

At this stage of your process, it is important to
address what I have found to be one of the most
common and pernicious problems barring full
access to a constant, satisfying, and lively sexual
connection. It is what I consider to be the *opposite* of connection and the *opposite* of desire—
and it is called **denial.**

When you say *no* to yourself and to your sexual needs, wants, dreams, fantasies, and pleasures, you are in essence setting up a chain of
events that systematically closes doors and
blocks access to a tremendous amount of feeling
and sensation inside you. You become impris-
oned in a four-by-four-foot-square cell of space
when, actually, you inhabit an entire mansion of
expression and possibility. Getting close and

connected involves learning to say *yes*. It's saying **yes** to your impulses and desires. It's saying **yes** to your wishes and dreams. It's giving yourself permission to be the *you* nobody knows.

Who is the sexual "you" that nobody knows? Who is the woman living silently inside you who is just dying for the opportunity to experiment, express, and explore every nook and cranny of her hot, dirty mind? If you stopped saying *no* to her and started saying *yes*, who would emerge? What would she look like? What would she do? What would she want right now? It's high time you found out.

"Wanting" Exercise #2

Go into your bedroom, bathroom, home office, or other private area and lock the door. Sit in a comfortable chair (or lie down on a couch or bed). Inhale through your nose as you slowly count to five. Count to five as you exhale through your mouth. Relax. Be present in your body. Close your eyes.

You're going to picture you and your partner together, beginning to make love. But things aren't exactly as they usually are because you have given your "body double" permission to take over. Who is your body double? She's the woman who says yes to your deepest, darkest, dirtiest sexual thoughts and feelings.

Now that you've made the "switch," where do you find yourself with your partner? Are you in the shower together?

In front of a roaring fire? In the backseat of a car? What are you wearing? It doesn't have to be thigh-high boots and crotchless panties (although that **does** sound pretty hot, doesn't it?). Maybe being a little teenybopper with pigtails, bobby socks, and white cotton panties turns you on. Relinquish control to your body double and let her take over; let yourself be a nonjudgmental observer and see where it takes you.

Now imagine what your twin is doing. Is she more aggressive than you are? More subservient? What form does that take? What does it involve? Does she vocalize more than you do? Does she moan, scream, whimper . . . ? Does she beg? How does she talk to your partner? What is she saying to him and how does she say it? What is she asking him to do? Is she using language that is different from yours? How does that make you feel?

It is perfectly natural for you to be feeling stimulated right now. Perhaps you are already masturbating. If so, good for you! You are embracing your "shadow self" and allowing her to connect you with parts of yourself that can help you experience the sexual awakening you long for.

Allow yourself at least fifteen minutes to fully observe your body double at play. When you're through, take a few minutes to record the experience in your journal.

Copy and write:

THE THING I FIND MOST EXCITING ABOUT MY BODY DOUBLE IS:

THE THING THAT SURPRISES ME MOST ABOUT MY
BODY DOUBLE IS:

THE THING THAT MADE ME MOST UNCOMFORTABLE
WAS:

THE THING(S) I MOST WANT TO WORK ON IS/ARE:

I hope that using the exercises and techniques
you discovered in this chapter as a means of fanning the flames of your sexual desire will become
as natural to you as saying *gesundheit* when someone sneezes. Why wait for more desire to find
you when you can so easily find more desire by
connecting to your own internal state of wanting?
Practicing these exercises and techniques is not
only a way to get yourself in "the mood" for sex.
Because they are so playful, so energizing, so
wild, and so creative, they get, and *keep* you, in
the mood for living!

7

Dreaming

i once worked with a woman who very much wanted to give her husband oral pleasure the way she had seen it done in several X-rated films. But every time she would take more than an inch or two of her husband's penis into her mouth. her throat would constrict and she would begin to gag. The situation was extremely frustrating and emotionally painful for both of them. After having ruled out the possibility of a past traumatic experience that could be responsible for her reaction, we continued to work on visualization techniques and the "inch-by-inch" approach. But progress was slow.

Then one afternoon she appeared at my office all smiles. I listened with fascination as she related to me a dream she had wherein she was able to perform fellatio on her partner with gusto and ease. She had fallen asleep the night before visualizing herself pleasing her partner with her mouth. In the dream, she was able to *feel* the way her throat could relax so that the gag response would not be triggered. Upon awakening, the dream was still vivid in her mind, and so was her belief in her ability to relax her throat and not panic. Feeling inspired and thoroughly optimistic, she immediately burrowed under the covers to test what she had learned from the dream. And her partner woke to a very pleasant dream of his own.

HARNESSING THE POWER OF EROTIC DREAMS

I believe that our dreams are much more than simply the by-products of our overstimulated imaginations, or the way our brains "clean house." I believe that dreams have the power to teach and transform us, and that they are willing to *cooperate* with our consciously stated requests, wishes, and desires.

What aspects of your own sexuality would you most like to change? Do you want to feel more comfortable in and proud of your own body? Maybe you would like to experience more frequent or powerful orgasms. Would you enjoy being more sexually expressive of your appreciation of and desire for your partner's body? Whatever it is you wish for, your dreams may hold the key.

"Dreaming" Exercise #1

Keeping in mind the aspects of yourself revealed to you by your "body double" in the previous chapter, take a moment to write down some of the ways in which you would like to effect a change in your sexuality:

Copy and write:

THE THING I WOULD MOST LIKE TO CHANGE ABOUT MY SEXUALITY IS:

DURING SEX, I WOULD LIKE TO BE ABLE TO:

I WISH I FELT MORE COMFORTABLE WITH:

In the weeks to come, you are going to ASK YOUR DREAMS TO SHOW YOU how you can change, and how to be more comfortable with things you wrote down on the list.

WEEK #1:

Every night before you go to sleep, concentrate on the first item on your list. PICTURE yourself enjoying the change in your sexuality that you desire. See yourself BEING the way you desire to be. Then, as you drift off to sleep, silently ASK your dreams to show you how you can effect the change you desire.

Be sure to keep a pad of paper and a pen by your bedside so that you can write down your dream upon waking. Every single time I have not written down a dream because it was so vivid I thought I would remember it, I have forgotten it.

You may have a dream you recognize as being relevant to your request the very first night. If after a week you **don't** feel as though you are getting a response to your request, you may want to:

A. make sure that you are repeating your request several times before you fall asleep;

B. ask that the dream be presented in a straightforward way you can understand;

C. ask that you remember your dream upon awakening.

Week #2

In week two, you are going to focus on the second item on your list. Every night before you go to sleep, you are going to visualize yourself DOING the thing you wish you could do during sex and you are going to ASK your dreams to show you how to accomplish it. If you hit a snag, follow the steps outlined above.

Week #3

In week three, you are going to focus on the third item on your list. As you fall asleep, visualize yourself at ease with the act you want to become comfortable with. Follow the same procedure as you did for weeks one and two.

If Albert Einstein could work out formulas for complex mathematical equations in his dreams, there is no reason why you can't work out your own personal formulas for erotic transformation while you sleep! If you can dream it, you can be it, do it, live it. You don't have to limit yourself to just your sexual issues; use this dreaming technique for *any* area in your life where you feel you are stuck and could use a nudge.

BRINGING YOUR DREAMS INTO YOUR REALITY

Coaxing your subconscious mind into having dreams that show you how to free and change your sexuality will do little good if you lose the content of those dreams moments after you wake. You need to be able to remember the details of those dreams and bring those dreams forward into the day with you. But how? Part of making a vital connection involves SLOWING DOWN, and one of the best places to begin slowing down is first thing in the morning, right after you wake up from a sexy dream.

When that alarm clock goes off in the morning, how many of you roll over, slap off the alarm or hit the snooze button, drift back to sleep, and then bolt out of bed at the last possible moment, completely jarring your senses and erasing *any* vestige of the dream you were having? We turn on the TV and gulp down a cup of coffee, thus giving ourselves no chance to "pan for gold" in the dreamscape from the night before.

As part of your program toward getting close and connected, I would like you to commit to a new STANDARD OPERATING PROCEDURE for waking up in the morning. Your new morning SOP will involve:

1. Training yourself to remain aware of the dream you have just had as you first wake up, instead of rushing to embrace the external reality of the day and letting the dream disappear.

2. Staying in bed, keeping your eyes closed, and wandering back into the content of the dream to prolong it for as long as possible (keeping the cameras rolling, so to speak).

3. Becoming the "director" of the extended dream footage—consciously trying to direct the action, having the dream turn out however you want it to.

4. Writing down as much of your dream as you can remember when you finally do open your eyes and leave your dream "trance."

Even if you drift back to sleep after hitting the snooze bar, take the few extra minutes before you bolt out of bed to remember and record your dreams. Remember: IF YOU DREAM IT, IT WILL COME, but first, you have to remember what you dreamed!

POWER DREAMING

You are probably already aware of the fact that some people in search of spiritual enlightenment hang crystals or pyramids over their beds because they believe that these objects have the power to raise their consciousness. The objects also serve as a focus for their attention as they drift off to sleep.

In keeping with this philosophy, here's a fun way to help lay the groundwork for a night of *sexual* enlightenment and sexually explicit dreaming.

"Dreaming" Exercise #2

Choose an object or item that represents the essence of sex to you. It can be your favorite dildo, your partner's sexy briefs, a catalog of sex toys and lingerie, a small piece of erotic sculpture, a primitive statue with a penis or vagina, or anything else of your choosing that puts you in a sexual frame of mind.

Place the item under your mattress. *This item is going to be your "totem"—a powerful symbol to organize your* sexual energy. *If you live by yourself, have no children, and rarely bring friends over on the spur of the moment, you might even want to hang your totem over your bed. You will **definitely** have a sexual thought, not to mention a gig-gle, every time you look at it. But a public display is not necessary. Kept under your mattress, the sexual totem will be out of sight, but it will not be out of mind.*

You will always know your sexual totem is there. *Whether you are thinking of it consciously or not, every time you get into, make up, or even just look at your bed, there is a part of you that will be aware of the sexual object you have placed just inches beneath you. Like a pyramid or a crystal, your object of power and enlightenment will work its magic on you at all hours of the day and night.*

Change your totem once a month. *Make it a game to find a new "object of desire" to spark your nocturnal activ-ity and inspire new and expansive sexual dreams. Keep it fresh!*

ALWAYS DREAMS, NEVER NIGHTMARES

As you begin to put energy into eliciting erotic dreams, there is a chance that some of the dreams you have will seem out of character, slightly bizarre, or over the top. Does this mean that the dream is a mandate that must be fol-lowed even though it might make you uncom-fortable? **Absolutely not.** Just because you dream of doing something doesn't mean that you have to do it, should do it, or have actually done it. If the dream was pleasurable for you and you were doing something you would never *dream* of doing in your waking life (making love to someone besides your partner, for example), it certainly is nothing to feel guilty about! Remember, it was only a dream.

One of the indications that you are having the type of dream the exercises in this chapter are designed to help you have is your enjoyment of its content, and the exciting and nonthreatening way in which the material shows up for you. Another indication is the sense of sexual exhilaration you are left with from the dream, even if the content is ambiguous or complex. But please note: If you find that you are consistently having dreams that are disturbing or upsetting to you, I would encourage you to engage a professional therapist who can help you understand the "what" and "why" of the material that is presenting itself.

DAYDREAMS COUNT, TOO

So many wonderful books have been written about the richness of women's erotic fantasies that most of us have become much more accepting of these "daydreams" we have. But what do you do with these daydream fantasies? Do you let yourself get lost in them, or are you embarrassed by their content and thus always fighting to push them out of your consciousness? Do you write them down, explore them in detail, and value their content, or do you tend to dismiss their value?

Many of us respect the powerful nature of the dreams we have while we sleep, yet we don't pay enough attention to the dreams we have when our eyes are wide open. Dreaming yourself into a sexual connection means giving *all* dreams equal weight, and that includes your daydreams.

"Dreaming" Exercise #3:
Open your journal to a clean page, then copy and complete the following:

MY THREE FAVORITE SEXUAL FANTASIES ARE:

1. _____
   _____
   _____

2. _____
   _____
   _____

3. _____
   _____
   _____

Over the next three days, set aside an hour each day to write out the details of each of these fantasies if you could bring them to life right now. Be very graphic and very elaborate, as if you were writing an erotic story or complex instructions for the making of a film. Talk about the lighting, the smells, the tastes, the textures, and, more than anything, the feelings—all of the things we have been focusing on in this book. Bring your fantasy to life on paper. This simple act of concretizing the workings of your imagination with pen and paper will help you acknowledge how fully sexual you are, and will bring you that much closer to making dreams come true. These are both your bedtime stories and your anytime stories. Read them again and again and let yourself feel the connection.

8
Words

When the seduction is complete, and it's time for making love, does the room get so silent that you could hear a pin drop? Are you a woman who believes that when it comes to lovemaking, "words only get in the way"? Does it seem strange to you to have a chapter devoted to "words" in a book about sexual connection? Then you are just the woman I need to talk to! Yes, sex is very much about touch and physical sensation. But add some scorching *verbal* stimulation to the mix and you start playing with an erotic fire that can very quickly get deliriously out of control!

I have a friend who would be the first to admit to being a "shrinking violet" when it comes to things of a sexual nature (not *all* of my friends are sex therapists or surrogates!). For her, sex was just something you had to keep your boyfriend happy. When it was particularly good, she enjoyed it just a little bit more than a nice back rub. She was aware from the books she read and the movies she saw that sex had the potential to be much wilder than anything she had experienced—but she didn't really believe it. She had no concrete experience to help her believe it. Until, that is, she met "the man with the golden tongue."

"The man with the golden tongue" did not earn this nickname because of his fondness for cunnilingus (not to say that's a bad thing either!). He earned this nickname because he said the sexiest, filthiest things to my friend when they made love. These things he said and the way he said them opened up her heart, supercharged her libido, and completely unleashed the sexual animal inside her. They seduced and shocked her, intoxicated and emboldened her, aroused and electrified her.

My friend the shrinking violet had never experienced sex like this before in her life. These words had her walking around in a perpetual state of arousal. She had orgasms with this man that left her gasping for breath. Sexually speaking, she was being reborn, all because of this man's ability to speak the unspeakable and teach her to do the same. In the end, it wasn't enough to sustain the relationship between them, but it opened my friend's eyes to a whole other dimension of sexual pleasure.

You, too, can learn to add this exciting dimension to your sex life. Do you have thoughts during sex that you keep to yourself? Phrases that pop into your mind that you dare not utter? Things that you would like to tell your partner but don't? Most of us do, and it's time to get the words off of the tip of your tongue and into your lover's ear.

"Words" Exercise #1
Pick a time when no one else is home. Go into your bedroom and lock the door. Get out your favorite dildo, vibrator, or combination of toys. Put on a sex video if you like. You may want to play some music if it makes you feel less self-conscious about making noise. Start to masturbate; as you do, START TALKING OUT LOUD. Begin by stating the obvious.

> *Start with:*
> *"My hand is moving back and forth."*
> *"My skin is so sensitive."*
> *"The vibrator is stimulating my clitoris."*
> *"The dildo is slippery and hard."*
> *"I can feel myself getting excited."*

> *Work up to:*
> *"That's so good."*
> *"You do that just right."*
> *"Don't stop."*
> *"Yes . . . yes . . ."*
> *"Ohhhh, yes!"*

Then:
"*I'm so wet.*"
"*Kiss my _____.*"
"*I need you to _____ me.*"
"*Your _____ is so _____.*"
"*I wish you could _____ me and _____ me at the same time.*"
"*_____ me now!*"
(Use your erotic imagination to fill in the blanks.)

And, finally, yelling:
"*Do it, do it, do it!*"
"*I'm going to explode!*"
"*Please don't stop, don't stop, don't stop!*"
"*I'm coming!*"

What I have written are only suggestions to get you started. What you say doesn't have to make sense, you don't have to be polite, and it's against the rules to censor yourself. Just let it fly. No one is around to hear you. Be so nasty you embarrass yourself. Get loud! Go completely overboard.

Are you excited? Very excited? Great! Keep talking until you have said every nasty thing you have ever thought of while making love. When you're through (and you have caught your breath!), write about it in your journal:

What pictures came into your head when you were talking dirty?

*What words and phrases **really** turned you on?*

Did anything turn you off?

Write down some of the words and phrases you'd like to say to your partner:

*What are some words and phrases you wish he would say to **you**?*

"Words" Exercise #2

*Repeat the steps you followed in "Words" Exercise #1, but this time, PLACE A TAPE RECORDER BY THE SIDE OF THE BED. You are going to record yourself talking out loud while you masturbate. Pretend you're with your partner. Give yourself the same level of freedom as you did the first time you practiced talking sexy. **Don't hold back**. Allow yourself to say everything that comes into your mind as you go from being mildly aroused, to being highly stimulated, to climaxing. Make sure you breathe, relax, and let go. Focus on turning **yourself** on with your words. Don't try to guess what will turn your partner on. You must trust that if **you** are genuinely turned on, he'll be turned on, so please your own ear first.*

HEARING IS BELIEVING

Label the tape words so you can identify it, and put it in a very private, very safe place. Then, the next time you masturbate, play the tape. How do you sound to yourself? Do you sound *connected* to your sexual core? If listening to yourself arouses you, then you were most likely connecting with your sexual essence. But if the tape leaves you cold, now try recording yourself again. Once you have made a tape you are satisfied with, keep it in a safe place for later use.

Please remember that when you talk dirty you aren't trying to be someone you're not. This is not about imitating something you once saw or trying to fulfill an image you think your partner has of you. **These exercises are about liberating the words that already exist within you.** All you are doing is giving them that proverbial first "inch" so that they will take you that extraordinary mile. If you would like to explore erotic verbalization to an even greater degree, my book *Talk Sexy to the One You Love* focuses exclusively on freeing the dirty words inside you.

WRITING AN OBSCENE LETTER

In the next exercise, I am going to ask you to write an obscene letter to the one you love. This is one of my favorites. The best part about writing this letter is that you never have to show it to your partner. In fact, I *recommend* that you don't. Like one of your "sexy secrets," the power of this exercise lies in its personal nature. Writing an obscene letter to your partner really revs up your sexual juices. It's like grabbing the end of a thunderbolt and then reaching out and touching your partner; it's completely electrifying!

"Words" Exercise #3
Open your journal to a clean page and begin writing an obscene letter to the one you love. Take your time. Be as graphic as possible. Leave no detail out.

Here is a sample:

> *Dear _____,*
> *I've been thinking about you all day long, and the way that I feel when we're naked and you're lying on top of me. I love running my fingers through your curly chest hair while I tease your hard nipples and softly bite at them with my teeth. My greatest pleasure is hearing you moan with passion and desire. I want to take your tongue deep into my mouth as I lightly stroke your gorgeous penis into a rock-hard state. . . .*

I would go on, but I'm starting to hyperventilate! I'm sure you get the picture and can take it from here. Write your letter all the way through to climax—both his and yours. Don't skimp on the details; talk about the special things he likes for you to do. Describe how you will lavish attention on the sensitive areas of his body that only you know about. Experiment with new vocabulary. Let the words flow.

It is my professional, instinctual, and educated guess that you will be ready for sex after writing this letter! You can write an obscene letter any time you feel that the flames of your desire need a little fanning. It is yet another way in which you can take more control of your sexual destiny. Since desire is a state of mind, think of writing an obscene letter to your partner as taking the express lane on the highway to Passion City, USA.

EROTIC AFFIRMATIONS

There are many books on the market today that provide daily meditations and affirmations especially for women. There are affirmations for women who work and have families, for women who want to deepen their spirituality, for teachers, for co-dependent women, and myriad other meditation books focusing on areas in which women want to effect change or bring peace into their lives. But where is the book of daily affirmations for women who want to get in touch with, stay in touch with, and increase their access to their most deeply sexual selves? Apparently, this is something you're going to have to write for yourself!

But before you begin to write your own custom-tailored sexy affirmations, there is something I would like you to think about. If you are what you eat, then even more so you are what you *think*. Descartes said, "I think, therefore I am." Dr. Barbara Keesling says that when it comes to sex, "Whatever I *think* I am, I am." Let me illustrate with two cases . . .

I'm sure that every woman reading this book knows at least one "Lola." By the current standards set forth by the American Medical Association, Lola is about thirty pounds overweight. If you happened to see Lola right as she got out of bed in the morning, you would probably describe her as average looking. But try telling any of this to *her*. Lola moves, walks, and talks with a sensual ease and grace. She "accentuates the positive" in her manner of dressing. Her sexy speaking voice always turns heads. She takes care with her hair and makeup. Men tend to describe her as "striking" and "hot." If you could read her mind, you would probably hear these thoughts: "I have a body built for sex"; "Any man is lucky to be with me"; "I have the loveliest breasts in the room"; "I have a deep capacity for sexual pleasure"; "I'm great in bed." It is obvious at first glance that Lola holds herself in high esteem and has a strong, vital connection to her erotic core.

And then there is "Mary." Mary would be considered pretty by many, and her measurements are technically ideal, but her slumped shoulders, closed expression, and lackluster presentation of herself make her easily forgettable. There is rarely a day when the clothes she is wearing wouldn't be completely appropriate on a man. She speaks so softly people always have to ask her to repeat herself. She cuts her own hair (badly) and basically walks around as if apologizing for taking up the space. Men tend to refer to her as "Mary who?" If you could read her mind you would probably hear thoughts like: "Everyone is more attractive than I am"; "What man would want me?"; "I'm terrible in bed—I had a boyfriend once who told me so"; "Men don't like to make love to me because I'm frigid." You can tell after several seconds in Mary's presence that she is a long way off from being connected to her erotic core.

As you can plainly see from these two examples (and probably already knew), **the only one whose truth matters is your own.** Since you are what you think you are, then it is crucial that you begin to take control of the thoughts that define the quality of your life as a sexual being, and the *words* that create these thoughts. As Descartes might have said, had he lived just a little longer: "I think I'm sexy, therefore I *am* sexy."

"Words" Exercise #4

In your sex goddess journal, copy the following:

WEEK #1

SUNDAY

MONDAY

TUESDAY

WEDNESDAY

THURSDAY

FRIDAY

SATURDAY

Repeat this again for week two. For each day of the week, write a sexual affirmation that is powerful to you and holds special meaning for you. For week one, all of the affirmations will start with the word "I." Make it one simple sentence that is easy to remember because you will be repeating the affirmation many times a day.

Some examples:
"I am in constant contact with my sexual self."
"I have an abundance of sexual energy."
"I say yes to my sexual thoughts and feelings."
"I am sexy right now, just as I am."
"I am a dynamic and exciting sexual partner."

"I get sexier every day."
"I accept great sex as one of the gifts of life."

During week two, your affirmations will focus more on parts and/or functions of your body.

For example:
"I can get sexually aroused at the drop of a hat."
"I have an extremely sensitive clitoris."
"I love having my _____ _____ed."
"My round bottom turns men on."
"I love to show off my _____."
"I'm an expert at _____."
"My partner loves to _____ me."
"I have a beautiful _____."
"My vagina feels sexy and wonderful."

Make up as many sexual affirmations as you like. You can focus on any aspect of your sexual self where you feel you need a change of perspective or an added boost. Now treat these affirmations the way you would treat any other. Make your sexy affirmation of the day a "mantra"—something you repeat over and over. Put Post-its in your glove compartment with your sexy affirmations on them. Create bookmarks (for home use only) with sexy affirmations written on them. Put sexy affirmations in your shoes, your wallet, your bra! Surround yourself with words that support your essence and your desire.

Very soon, having only *positive* thoughts about your body and your sexuality will become second nature to you. When that happens, you will experience a fundamental shift in thought, attitude, and behavior that will be nothing short of profound in the impact it will have on your life both in and out of bed! When it comes to sex, words don't get in the way. Words *are* the way. So remember, THINK SEXY!

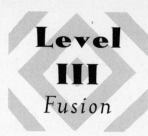

Level III
Fusion

You came to this book with the desire to build a more powerful sexual connection with your partner. But the first thing you discovered was that you had to create a more powerful connection with yourself. You've already worked very hard, had some fun, too, and overcome many barriers to achieve a level of sexual connectedness, sensitivity, freedom, and responsiveness you've never known before. Gone is the lethargic, unresponsive woman who first picked up this book; in her place stands someone who is ready, willing, and able to access the most sizzling hot realms of her sexual being and bring that part of herself into her relationship with her partner.

And now it's fusion time—time to complete the connection. Your solo journey has ended; you are ready to come together with the one you desire and discover, as a couple, a whole new world of sexual expression and erotic delight. You have everything you need to start enjoying the most erotic, electric, tantalizing sexual connection you have ever known. You are fully prepared for the most exciting part of the adventure. So what are you waiting for? Let's get busy!

9

Asking

i've talked a fair amount about my professional experience in this book, but now that you are ready to fully incorporate your partner into the program, I want to share something a little more personal. I love it when my partner asks me to do things for him when we are making love; I feel so close to him when he does. I know that he has opened his sexual core to me. I feel he is trusting me with his most intimate needs and desires; it also gives me pleasure to know that I am pleasing him to the utmost. Most of all, it lets me know that it's okay for me to ask *him* for the things I need from him.

You may not be used to asking your partner for what you want and need, but the time has come for that to change. It's time to put aside the notion once and for all that the man in your life can read your mind. Sexual connection demands sexual communication. You're in a relationship, not the army; so DO ASK and DO TELL your partner your deepest desires. I'm not suggesting that you try to share this all in one night; that would be overwhelming to anyone. But you owe it to yourself and to your partner to be true to the very sexual "you" you've worked so hard to discover. Making a powerful sexual connection means making a commitment to being honest with yourself and your loved one about who you are and what you want and need. And the time for that commitment is now.

Understand that this doesn't mean that your partner has to comply just because you have asked; he has to feel free to say *no* if he is uncomfortable with your request—that's how it works in a democracy. But you may be surprised by how much your partner is willing to do, as well as the number of requests you receive in turn from him once you open the door.

This isn't a chapter about talking dirty (though we'll do a little of that, too), it's a chapter about talking straight. The time for beating around the bush has come and gone; if you want your "bush" to be "beat," then, girlfriend, that's exactly what you're going to ask for!

ASKING HIM IN

Did you show the man in your life this book when you first started reading it? If not, ASK him to look at it now. The best way for you and your partner to "get on the same page" is for him to become familiar with the material in this book. Want to make it fun? **Take turns reading aloud to each other at bedtime.** You can read the whole book, or pick highlights. Your partner will probably marvel at everything you have done to enhance the quality of your sexual relationship. You may find yourselves reminiscing a little bit, remembering times when you sexually attacked him for no apparent reason!

If you have any anxiety about sharing certain aspects of your newly "hatched" sexual self with your partner, now is the time to discuss it. Let your partner know about any fears of rejection you may have and how vulnerable you would be to any criticism or negative comments he may make about the process you have just completed. If your lover understands that everything you have done up to this point has been to bring you here, to this moment, where you are on the brink of sharing new heights and depths of sexual passion with him, I trust he will do his best to meet you with love, acceptance, and enthusiasm.

Don't be surprised if your partner has some anxiety of his own. He may feel that a lot is being asked of him in the pages ahead—he may even feel it's a bit too much. I hope this will not be the case. But if your loved one does express

anxiety or unwillingness in this way, be patient
with him. He may have been perfectly satisfied
with your sex life before and see no need for
change. Take it step by step, day by day. Your
partner may simply need some time to get used
to the idea of things being a little (or a lot) different. If he can see and appreciate just how
important it is for you to feel more connected to
him, he will be motivated to join you in many of
the playful, extremely sensual, and incredibly
bonding exercises that I have designed for your
mutual enjoyment and pleasure.

A QUICK, BUT CRUCIAL, REALITY CHECK

This is the very late twentieth century, and I
hope that you are already so informed and
responsible that my discourse on using condoms
and practicing safe sex, if you have not been in a
committed relationship with your partner for
very long, will be entirely unnecessary.

HOWEVER, allow me to reiterate: NO
GLOVE, NO LOVE; and regular blood tests
are a *must*. Don't take chances with your health.
These exercises are intended for couples who
have been together long enough to know and be
comfortable with one another's histories. If you
and your partner don't fit into that category, give
yourselves the chance to by protecting your-

selves in the meantime. NO exceptions, NO excuses. Now, on with the show!

WHAT YOU SHOULD KNOW ABOUT THE COUPLES' EXERCISES:

Be sure to read through all of the couples' exercises at least once before you begin. Here are some basic things you and your partner need to know about each of these exercises before you get started:

- *An exercise does not have to lead to sex unless that is specifically stated.*
- *Orgasm is not the goal unless that is specifically stated.*
- *Some physical activity is usually involved.*
- *More than anything, the exercise should leave you with a feeling of energy and vitality.*
- *There is nothing competitive about it.*
- *If you can't finish the exercise, don't start (you must agree on a time that is good for both of you, when you can fully devote yourselves to the activity, AND you must set aside the appropriate amount of time needed to complete the exercise).*
- *If you're feeling pressured, don't continue. Your primary goal always is to enjoy yourself.*

Now get ready, because here they come. Whole new ways of touching, teasing, loving, seducing, kissing, and hugging are just pages away. You are a very special person to have made it this far in your quest for sexual connection, and I commend you. You have always deserved the immense joy and sexual ecstasy that is coming your way, and now you have earned it, too! Being sexually connected isn't strange and it isn't a fluke; it is the way each and every one of us is *supposed* to be. So embrace the connection!

RETURN TO THE LOVING TOUCH

The first thing you are going to ASK your partner to do is to simply *watch* as you give yourself a full-body loving touch. This may be the first time your partner has ever watched you touch yourself and he may get very excited, particularly if it brings out the voyeur in him; but it's important that he allow you to complete your loving touch uninterrupted. The purpose of this exercise is for him to become familiar with this way of touching and to learn from you exactly where you enjoy being touched most. How is he going to know which areas are your most responsive? That's simple. You're going to SHOW and TELL him, of course!

"Asking" Exercise #1

Get your oils and lubricants. Lie naked, within close prox-imity to your lover; make sure he can see what you're doing. Take as many of your deep, slow, sensual breaths as you need to relax. Close your eyes. ASK him if he is ready. Now begin a slow, sensual caress. You're probably going to feel a little more "amped" because of the presence of your lover, so pay attention to your speed. If you find yourself rushing, breathe in slowly, breathe out slowly, then cut your speed in half. Talk to your partner. TELL him when you are touch-ing an **area** that is particularly sensitive. SHOW him how you enjoy being touched there. TELL him which areas **aren't** particularly responsive. Touch yourself from the tips of your ears to the tops of your toes; let your partner know how everything feels along the way.

Give yourself a full genital touch as well. DON'T STOP TALKING. Keep breathing slowly, fully, and deeply. ASK your partner if he can see the way you are touching yourself. ASK him if there is something he wants to see again. TELL him what feels especially good. This isn't the time to masturbate in front of your partner—I promise, you **will** get the chance. For now, ASK, SHOW, and TELL; give your lover the deluxe "guided tour" to the body you've discovered anew.

When you're through, talk to your partner about the experience. How did watching you make him feel? How did touching yourself in front of him make you feel? What, if anything, felt uncomfortable to either of you? What turned you on the most? Is this something you would enjoy repeating?

This is the kind of talk you should have with your loved one after *every* exercise. Try not to leave issues or questions dangling between you; you want to clear the decks before moving on to each new exercise.

ASKING TO GET CLOSER

Since you have all of the experience (by now, you're practically an expert!), you're going to give your partner his first full-body loving touch. The whole thrust of this exercise is GETTING YOUR PARTNER'S PERMISSION to touch him and explore his body in ways you never have before. It's about gaining his trust and making a bond. It's about *asking* to be close to him.

"Asking" Exercise #2
Ask your partner to undress and lie down on a towel on the floor or on the bed. Lead him through a few relaxing sensual breaths. Warm the massage oil between the palms of your hands, then apply it to his body. Ask him to close his eyes. Sit or kneel by his side. Starting with his face, give your partner the same slow, light touch that you use on yourself.

You are focusing on the way your partner's skin feels under your fingertips, and on keeping your pace **slow**. He is concentrating on taking slow, deep breaths, and on fully experiencing the sensation of your touch on his skin. He is also making mental notes of what feels especially good to him, and any areas that are particularly unresponsive.

Move down your lover's body to the genitals. Keep your touch light; again, you are not going to masturbate him. Simply explore his genitals with your fingertips. If he gets an erection, so much the better, but continue your light, slow touch. Go all the way down his legs to his toes. Ask him to turn over. Apply more oil and work your way up to the top of his head on the back side of his body. Don't ignore his scalp and his ears.

Let him lie still for as long as he wants to when you are finished, then TALK about the experience as you did after the first exercise.

I hope your first couple's loving touch leaves you feeling loving and close to each other, It is something you can return to whenever the two of you want to relax and feel especially close.

But now it's time for you to ASK your partner to explore and learn your body. It's time for him to try his loving touch on you and begin putting everything he has been discovering in these first few exercises into practice.

"Asking" Exercise #3

Ask your partner to apply the oil to you just as you did to him. **Remember to breathe fully and deeply.** Now ask him to begin his touch. Since this is his first time, you may need to let him know if he needs to lighten his touch, or slow down. How does it feel to finally have your partner's fingers touch you in the way that has become so familiar to you? Open your legs so your lover can see **all** of you. Enjoy the sensations that come from being lightly stroked in this way.

If necessary, you can remind your partner that the genital touch is to remain **light** and sensuous, not forceful or intentionally sexual. He is feeling the textures, shapes, and sizes, not endeavoring to make you come. But DON'T distract him or burden him during his first loving touch by telling him what feels good or what doesn't feel good. Just make mental notes so you can talk about it later.

After you have been touched all over, front and back, lie still and let the feelings linger. Now you can let your lover know where his touch felt particularly good. Ask him what it was like for him to touch you in this way. Thank him for joining you, and get ready to ask for **more**.

ASKING ALL THE RIGHT QUESTIONS

I think the PC muscle is one of the most important muscles a woman can develop, but the *most* important muscle, in my opinion, is the "asking" muscle. And we're going to continue flexing this muscle and building its strength with the next exciting partner exercise: "Three Questions."

Three Questions is a hot, hot game that forces you to ask for *exactly* what you want from your partner. You only get to ask for three things in your alotted time, so you must be extremely specific in your requests. Your requests can involve something you want your partner to do to you, or it can be something you want to do to your partner. However, your partner has the right to refuse your request, no questions asked (as do you when it's his turn to do the asking). If he says, "I'm not comfortable with that right now," respect that and ask for something else. You are not at fault for asking, and he is not at fault for declining. Move on; hopefully he will choose to talk about what it was that made him uncomfortable after the exercise is over.

Your request doesn't necessarily *have* to be sexual; you may just wish to be held, or be given a massage. You may want your partner to bathe you, or to suck your toes, or to bring you ice cream. Start with something simple and comfortable and expand from there. You may find your request leads you to the bedroom, the bathroom, or the backseat of a car. It's entirely up to you. Just

be certain to agree ahead of time with your partner to make Three Questions a "neutral zone"
where all judgment gets suspended and you get to
let it "all hang out."

I think you will find that Three Questions
expands your sexual comfort zone with your
partner and makes it much easier for you to bring
more of your sexual/sensual nature into bed on a
regular basis. And, believe it or not, it will really
help you with your communication skills—particularly your ability to express your immediate
needs clearly and directly. Some of my clients
become so fond of this game that it becomes an
integral part of the way they make love all the
time. Why? Because THERE IS SOMETHING
VERY SEXY ABOUT ASKING AND GET-
TING PERMISSION FROM YOUR PART-
NER. Try it now, and see.

"Asking" Exercise #4

*For the first half of this exercise, you will be the "asker" and
your partner will be the "doer." Halfway through, you will
switch roles. Allow thirty to forty-five minutes for each partner.*

*As the asker, you get to ask for up to three things that you
would enjoy doing to your partner, or having your partner
do to you. Before you make a request of your partner, close
your eyes and think a moment about what you **really want
to have happen**. What would really feel good to you now?*

You don't have to worry about forcing your partner to do something that he doesn't want to do because he always has the option of saying **no**. So ask for whatever you want.

Be very specific in your request. For example, don't say "Take off all your clothes" when what you really mean is "Do a striptease for me." This is a chance to really sharpen those communication skills.

It is between you and your partner as to how long any one activity will go on. But if the doer is ready to quit before you are, then it's time to quit. Obviously, certain activities will be ruled by physical limitations (Can't you just hear it? "Honey, I love you, but I can only squat for so long!").

If the asker's request involves doing something to the other partner, then the request must be phrased: "May I please____(fill in the blank)?" You can do whatever you want *to* **yourself** while your request is being fulfilled (for example, you can masturbate while your partner is stripping for you), but ANY KIND OF TOUCHING OF YOUR PARTNER REQUIRES GETTING PERMISSION FIRST, AND COUNTS AS ONE OF YOUR REQUESTS!

If your request isn't being fulfilled in quite the way you had imagined it, you can opt to gently instruct your partner, either verbally or through physical demonstration. But in this game, give A's for effort, and NEVER LET YOUR REQUESTS SOUND LIKE DEMANDS. I'm sure your partner can tell the difference between a little playful dominant behavior on your part and genuine belligerence; an

impatient or demanding tone is one sure way to take all of
the fun out of Three Questions, and this is a game that you
will want to play for years and years to come.

ASKING TO TALK SEXY TO
THE ONE YOU LOVE

This is a subject that is near and dear to my
heart, which is probably why I can't stop writing
about it. We've talked about this already in
"Words." But we need to talk about it here as
well because it is such an important component
of making a close connection with your partner.

As I said at the beginning of this chapter, making
a sexual connection demands sexual communication, and I know of no more direct and exhilarating
way of sexually communicating than talking sexy to
your lover when you are making love. If you have
ever disobeyed the instructions on a can of char-
coal lighter fluid and squirted a little extra on
already lit coals, then you can conjure up the explosive mental image of what a few well-timed, well-
chosen words can do in the midst of sex.

When it is rooted in passion, sex talk acts as an
accelerator, unleashing a little atomic bomb of
energy when it hits the air. As we all know, atomic
energy is strong stuff, so it should not be brought
into the bedroom without your partner's previous

knowledge and consent. Not only might he wonder where you got the plutonium from, but if he
isn't wearing the proper protection, you could
vaporize him! So you need to have a conversation
(if you are reading this chapter together, you've
got a nice head start) with your partner telling
him of your desire, and letting him know that you
wish to tell him what's going through your beautiful dirty little mind when you are making love.
Chances are, it *will* be okay with him. In fact, you
will probably wind up with a recruit on your
hands; let's hope so!

Do you remember the tape you made back in
"Words" (Chapter 8)? Well, get it out of the
safety deposit box where you've been hiding it,
because it's time to let your lover know just what
a smooth and talented talker you really are.

"Asking" Exercise #5

*Close and lock your bedroom door, undress, and join your
partner in bed. Although the follow-up portion of this exercise ("Asking" Exercise #6) will involve sexual activity,
"Asking" Exercise #5 should be approached in a nonsexual
manner. You can lie down together if you like, but save your
lovemaking for later; the tape will require your undivided
attention.*

*Tell your partner about the tape that you made in
"Words." Now ASK him if you can play the tape for him*

*while you are here together in bed. Let him know that it was **him** you were thinking about while you were masturbating and talking out loud. Tell him that the things he will hear you saying on the tape are the things you would like to begin saying when you are in bed together. Explain that you have no expectations that he will respond in kind (although I'm assuming you would love it if he did!).*

Give your partner a pad of paper and a pencil. As he listens to the tape, ask him to write down any phrases or words that make him uncomfortable (if any). He is also welcome to write down all the words and phrases that he especially likes, too.

When the tape has ended, ask your partner how listening to you talk dirty makes him feel. Listen carefully to what he has to say. There's no point in asking if you're not listening to the answers.

If your partner immediately answers you with his mouth, lips, hands, and other body parts, you know you're getting an unequivocal "thumbs up." But if his answer is a little more restrained, try not to be disappointed. Do your best not to take personally any reserve on his part. You've just completed a course that has torn down many barriers and erased a lot of your sexual taboos; he hasn't. It may be necessary for you to introduce sexy language into your lovemaking slowly and gradually. If your partner has never heard you

utter a single dirty word during sex and now
you're stringing them together in a way that
would get you instantly hired on any 976 line, he
may need some time to get used to the new you.
No problem. You've got nothing but time. And
the next exercise will help accelerate his process.

"Asking" Exercise #6

*Rewind, then replay the tape you made in "Words." This
time, you're going to make love while the tape is playing.
Your heightened state of arousal from already hearing the
tape once, and your comfort from "breaking the ice," should
help melt away any residual unease.*

*Try echoing yourself as you make love. That is, repeat
after yourself the words you are saying on the tape. If the
"hottest" language on the tape proves to be a little too
intense for either of you at this point, then stick with
"medium-hot" phrases like:*

- *It feels so good when you do that.*
- *I love it when you touch me there.*
- *I'm so excited.*
- *Ohhhhhhh. Oooooooo.*
- *Yes, lover. Yes, yes, yes.*

*Just be sure to talk; say **something**. Let your partner get
used to hearing your voice and saying what is on your mind
and in your heart. Pretty soon, he won't remember a time*

when you didn't. He may even soon surprise you with a few words of his own!

In this chapter you learned to ASK directly for what you want so that you could both give *and* receive more when you are making love with your partner. And I'm sure both you and your partner are already feeling the difference in your emotional *and* sexual connection. Fusion begins when we break down barriers and begin to reveal our true desires through the honest process of asking. And it strengthens as we continue to ask, continue to risk, and delight in the feelings of having our partners respond to our honesty.

10

Surrender

What images does the word "surrender" conjure up for you? Do you picture someone backed into a corner, surrounded by federal marshals, being forced to come out with his hands up? That's what I feel like I'm encountering sometimes from my clients, both male and female, when I first introduce the concept of surrender. As with many sexual issues, the waters swirling around the concept of surrender have grown quite muddy. So let's take a look at what *I* mean when I speak of sexual surrender between you and your partner. First, let's look at what surrender *isn't*:

- *To surrender does not mean that you are weak.*
- *To surrender does not mean to abandon your own needs, principles, or morals in order to please your partner.*

- *To surrender does not mean that you remain the subservient partner in the bedroom for the rest of your life.*
- *To surrender is not an acknowledgment that one sex is better than the other.*

Now let's look at what surrender *is*:

- *To surrender is to be confident enough in your own power to be powerless for a while.*
- *To surrender is to trust enough in your partner to let him/her be in complete sexual control sometimes.*
- *To surrender is to trust enough in yourself to let down the gates that are barring you from experiencing the full range of your own sexuality.*
- *To surrender is to accept.*
- *To surrender is to serve.*
- *To surrender is to trust.*

In what places within yourself are you still holding on to concepts, judgments, or fears that repress you and keep you out of a full sexual connection with yourself and with your partner? This is the chapter where you are going to root them out, open them up, and let them go. It is time for both of you to lay down your arms, put down your dukes, and tear down the dam. It is time for you to surrender.

THE PEDI-"CURE"

Besides your genitals, is there anywhere on your body that is as sensitive or feels as vulnerable as your feet? It is no accident that the one area of weakness and vulnerability in one of the greatest characters in Greek mythology was located at his feet, his Achilles heel. There are more nerve endings in the feet than there are anywhere else, and the science of reflexology is based on the supposition that these nerve endings lead to every organ in the body.

On a more primal level, to place your feet in another's hands is an act of supreme trust and surrender. Some of the worst tortures ever devised involve the feet. Conversely, pleasant stimulation of the feet can produce some of life's most sublime physical sensations.

To minister to someone's feet is also an act of *deference* and surrender; it is a wonderful way to serve, connect with, relax, and please your partner. And that is why we're going to begin this chapter with a footbath. Giving your partner a footbath will not only increase the sense of intimacy between you, it will also help your partner feel more amorous by relaxing him (and later, you) at the end of a stressful day, and allowing him to shift his focus to you.

For the first exercise you will need:

1. a small basin (tub) or a dishpan large enough to place both of your partner's feet in at the same time

2. liquid soap or bath bubbles

3. body lotion or cream

4. two towels

"Surrender" Exercise #1

Fill the basin with enough warm water to reach up to your partner's ankles. Have your partner sit on a sofa or in a comfortable chair. Pick up his feet, one at a time, and place them into the tub of warm water. Drizzle enough of the liquid soap or bath bubbles into the water to make it feel soapy and slippery.

Working on one foot at a time, begin lightly stroking the top and sides of your lover's foot. As in the loving touch series of exercises, touch for your own pleasure. In many ways, this exercise should be as pleasurable for you as it is for your partner. Go very slowly. Try to feel every ridge and curve.

*After lightly stroking the entire surface for several minutes, increase your pressure and begin to massage the foot. Don't use **too** much pressure; this is a sensuous massage,* *not a therapeutic one. Just think of yourself as gently relaxing the muscles under your fingers. Massage each individual toe, between the toes, and the tendon just above the heel, too. After about ten minutes of massage on the first foot, switch to the other and repeat the same procedure.*

When both feet have been stroked and massaged, take one foot out of the bath and place it in a fluffy towel. Pat the foot dry. Massage the cream or lotion into the top and bottom of the foot, the ankle, and the toes. Dry and repeat with the other foot.

You will feel gratified as you watch the tension and stress level in your partner go down, allowing his desire and libido to rise. And remember, turnaround is fair play. Now that you have given your partner such a pleasurable demonstration of how it is done, next time switch roles. It's *your* turn to surrender your feet and his turn to surrender his power by giving you a loving footbath. I wouldn't be surprised if a footbath quickly becomes one of the favorite ways for both of you to give and receive pleasure. In fact, it may just prove to be the Achilles heel in both of you.

MORE TO SHOW AND TELL

Being the sexually connected vixen that you are, you may be miles ahead of me and have already taken your partner by the hand and led him into the wonderful world of sex toys and paraphernalia. But if you haven't, this is the part where you get to show and tell. If you've enjoyed playing with your toys in the past, just wait until you put them in the hands of your lover. Wow, are *you* in for a treat!

Presumably, your partner has read enough of this book to know that you have incorporated the use of toys into your solo sex life, so that he will not be in complete shock when you invite him to join you in your play. If, for some reason, your partner has not read that portion of this book, please read it with him now before you proceed with this exercise. You will possibly prevent a world of confusion and hurt feelings by doing so.

Why am I putting show and tell in the chapter on surrender?

Because it is yet another door you are opening, another border you are crossing, in order to more fully connect with your sexual partner. Allowing your man to join you in your use of toys requires your willingness to give up control, as well as showing a lot of trust. It is a profound, and profoundly pleasurable, way to wave the white flag.

Before you begin the next exercise, one thing you need to establish very clearly with your partner is that sex toys never have been and never will be a replacement for, or an improvement on, making love with him. If anything, the toys that you have been experimenting with have already helped you plumb new depths of sexual pleasure with *him*.

Which of your toys will you be "showing" and "telling"? That's up to you. Perhaps one vibrator and your favorite dildo would be a good place to start. It can't hurt to save a few of your other surprises for next time. But if you know that your partner is more adventurous, and if he's begging to see everything you've got, then by all means let him see everything you've got!

"Surrender" Exercise #2

Agree to set aside at least an hour with your partner for this exercise. Once you are in bed with your partner, explain to him that first you are simply going to SHOW him how you use your toys so that he will have a sense of the speeds, pressures, and movements that feel best to you.

Starting with the dildo, begin by showing your partner how much lubricant you put on it. Demonstrate the various ways you can play with the dildo before it even enters you, like rubbing your inner and outer lips with it, or making lazy circles on your clitoris. When you and he are both comfortable, let your partner "take the reins." Loosen your tongue, because you're going to be doing a lot of talking as you TELL your partner what feels good, where and why.

Let your partner know when you want him to ease the

dildo inside you. Breathe deeply and relax into the sensa-
tion of the dildo being manipulated by your lover's hand.
Since this will be a very new experience for him, give your
partner lots of positive reinforcement. Let him know that
what he's doing is extremely pleasurable to you. If neces-
sary, show your partner how you stroke yourself with the
dildo. Try putting your hand over his and let him feel what
it feels like as you please yourself with the stroke for a while.
Remove your hand and continue to give your lover positive
feedback and encouragement.

Don't put pressure on your partner or on yourself to
have an orgasm. *That's not fair to either of you. The goal*
here is to relax, explore, have fun, and feel good—for **both**
of you. If you put pressure on your lover to "perform," he
could feel so overwhelmed by the entire experience that he'll
never want to repeat it. I won't be at all surprised if you do
have an orgasm. But it shouldn't be a requirement for this
exercise.

You can introduce all of your toys to your partner using
this same procedure. First show him how you use the item
on yourself, then let him use it on you, guiding his hand
with yours, if necessary, so that he can get a feel for what
you like.

When it comes to sex, practice makes pleasurable. In the next exercise you and your partner
get to log in more playtime, this time with an
added twist. This exercise asks that you let go

even more into trust, because you will be *blind-folded* for the duration.

"Surrender" Exercise #3
Set aside at least forty-five minutes for this couple's exercise. Raid your "pleasure chest" and have your dildos, vibrators, and lubricants within easy reach. Have your lover tie the blindfold securely over your eyes. You and your partner are going to play hide-and-seek using the toys on hand. Some of the toys will wind up "hiding" inside you, while with others your partner is going to seek out the most sensation-filled spots on your body he can find.

This is not the time to give instructions; **unless your partner is doing something that is uncomfortable to you, remain silent** *(although it is perfectly okay to moan your brains out). Give your lover the opportunity to explore and experiment freely, and give yourself the opportunity to let go, give up control, and surrender to the excitement of not knowing what is going to come next.*

ARE YOU READY TO BE THE MAN IN BED?

Admit it; you got a little shiver up your spine reading the title of this section, didn't you? You can't hide it from me, I've seen too many eyes light up when I ask this question. We're going to ignore all of the deep psychological interpretations that so many would be tempted to cast on this. We're also going to ignore any political (or politically incorrect) overtones that some might want to assign. It's really very simple: Playing the man's part in bed for once can be very exciting. And fun, too! There's nothing sinister or unhealthy about it. It's an opportunity to walk a mile in your partner's shoes, as well as a chance to gain more insight into yourself.

Just as an actor can learn truths about herself by playing someone else, so can you learn truths about who you are as a woman by immersing yourself in the role of the man. Being the man means getting in touch with your power. Being the man means *surrendering* to the desire and curiosity that exist inside you to know what exercising that power feels like. For your partner, allowing you to be the man means putting aside his own power for a while and *surrendering* to yours. For him, allowing you to be the man means relinquishing control and letting you make love to him.

Sexually speaking, what else does "being the man" mean to you? Do you know? Take a minute to explore the concept fully. Get out your notebook and write:

TO BE THE MAN IN BED MEANS TO:

WHAT'S EXCITING TO ME ABOUT PLAYING THE MAN IS:

MY FEARS ABOUT PLAYING THE MAN ARE:

Are you surprised by any of your answers?

BRINGING OUT THE MAN IN YOU AND SURRENDERING THE WOMAN

Are you a gentle and sensitive lover? Or are you a bit of a brute? Maybe you're a little of both. What kind of a man *are* you? You're about to find out.

This next exercise will definitely require a conversation between you and your partner before you embark on it. Talk to your partner about any fears you might have. Decide ahead of time just how far you're both comfortable going in your role reversals. In your role as the man, do you want to wear different clothes? Walk differently? Talk differently?

Does the thought of wearing a strap-on penis excite you? Is your partner open to that? And what about him? Is there anything he'd like to do differently? Any props he would like to use?

Somehow, I doubt that the sight of your partner in a flimsy negligee will stimulate anything but a fit of the giggles. But I could be wrong, and if it works for both of you, roll with it.

"Surrender" Exercise #4

Start by undressing your lover. Have him sit on the edge of
the bed so that you can stand over him. Take your time with
each button, if that's your style. Or tear at his clothes if
you're that kind of man. Play with your partner's "breasts."
Lick and suck on his nipples.

Try not to do anything that will ruin the illusion for you
that you are the man. For example, don't call your partner
"pretty" if it seems silly to you. Instead say, "This is pretty,"
or, "I like the way this looks." How does the man in you
talk? What does his voice sound like? What is he saying?
Although you're playing a game, the more seriously you take
your roles, the more you'll both get out of it.

Are you fantasizing that you have a penis? Do you
want him to stroke it or suck it? Tell him. Or, if you're the
more brutish type, simply cradle your lover's head in your
hand and bring his face to your groin. Move your hips back
and forth in a "mannish" manner.

To simulate the act of penetration and experience the
feeling of dominance that accompanies it, you can "mount"
your partner from behind with him on all fours. Rub and
"thrust" against him and stimulate him with your vibrator
as you masturbate him (or he masturbates himself).

Are you still whispering sweet nothings? Or are you getting
down and dirty and tapping into a place in yourself you never
knew existed? As long as you're both enjoying yourselves,
there's no reason to stop, no reason to hold back. You may even
want your lover to affirm it for you: Ask him, "Who's the
man?" He replies, "You're the man." Damn right.

Did you enjoy that? I'm sure this exercise will generate a lot of discussion between you and your partner afterward. I stand in admiration of what a loving and trusting couple you must be to have completed this level of surrender. I hope that these challenging exercises, along with all of the exercises that await you just ahead in "Loving," will add greatly to your wealth of love, trust, intimacy, and knowledge.

11

Loving

the most powerful connection we can make with a loving partner is the connection we make through intercourse. Yet I have asked you to work through ten chapters—including two devoted entirely to couples' exercises—before finally arriving at the chapter that focuses specifically on intercourse. This, in a book by a sex therapist who is completely devoted to renewing, refreshing, and reviving your sexual connection with your partner. Maybe that seems strange to you, but as Pee Wee Herman used to say, "I *meant* to do that!" Yes. The delay has been completely intentional.

Why have I asked you to wait so long? Because I will not rush to intercourse. Not personally, and not professionally. Not as a lover, not as a therapist, not when I acted as a professional sex surrogate, and not as a writer. Look at all of the acts of love you have completed as a part of this program, both by yourself and with your partner, that have *not* focused on intercourse. And yet they were very sexual, very sensual, and very exciting. Some, overwhelmingly so.

To many, intercourse is the big brass ring on the merry-go-round; it's the pot of gold at the end of the rainbow, it's Xanadu. Listen, I don't disagree; intercourse is the most physically intimate act two adults can share, and I look forward to showing you in the pages to come how it actually has the power to transform. What tends to happen, though, in our "hurry-up-Jay Leno-is-about-to-come-on-world," is that in our rush to "get it on" and "get off" we effectively whiz by an entire **world** of feeling, connection, and soul communion with our mates.

This attitude toward sex reminds me of the way some people refer to any city that isn't on one of the coasts as "fly-over country." Just as the interior of an entire nation is not "fly-over country," neither should the stops along the way to intercourse and orgasm (your bodies, subtle sensations, shared moments) be so easily dismissed. In the same way that human beings only utilize 10 percent of their brain capacity, we also tend to tap into only a fraction of the amazing power, energy, and love we could be experiencing when we make love.

So what's the answer? Am I implying that you have to set aside hours and hours every time you have sex? Absolutely not. I'm a realist, and I live in the world, too. What I *am* saying is that by SLOWING DOWN, by not necessarily rushing to intercourse and rushing *through* intercourse, by giving yourselves *a real chance to experience each other*, you will increase your connection to your partner tenfold and change forever what you think of as making love.

FEELING THE CONNECTION

Now that we have fully attended to so many of the aspects of the sensuality and sexuality that lead up to intercourse, we are free to explore the act itself. All of the exercises in this chapter begin at the point of intercourse. This doesn't mean that *you* have to begin there. You have now learned so many ways to "begin" from the moment you wake up in the morning (and even when you prepare for sleep the night before). But however you choose to prepare for these exercises—whether you use them in conjunction with other exercises or just "jump right in" where these exercises begin—the "work" focuses solely on intercourse.

Although intercourse allows two people to get physically closer than any other act, physical proximity doesn't always translate into a feeling of *connection*. In fact, if you have intercourse before having established a sense of connection with your partner, a feeling of *dis*-connection can actually be exacerbated. One good way to reestablish a sense of intimacy with your partner is to slow down the act of intercourse itself. And, as you will see in this first intercourse exercise, **the best way to reestablish a feeling of connection with your partner during intercourse is to come to a complete standstill.**

"Loving" Exercise #1
Allow fifteen minutes for this exercise. Have lots of lubricant on hand.

Begin with several slow, sensual breaths, taken together, to the count of five (five seconds inhaling, five seconds exhaling). Breathe in through the nose, and out through the mouth. You can lie side by side on your backs holding hands, or cuddled like two "spoons," or one partner can lie on top of the other so that you can feel the breath moving into and out of your bodies. Choose what feels best for you.

When you are both feeling relaxed and centered, slather some lubricant on your lover's penis. He can put some lubricant on your vagina at the same time. Slowly, sensually masturbate your partner just until he is hard enough to enter you; a full erection is not necessary.

Once your partner is inside you, wrap your arms around one another and gaze into each other's eyes. DON'T MOVE and DON'T SPEAK. Let the energy that normally would be expelled through movement and speech build and flow between you.

Your partner's erection will probably go up and down.

That is fine. In fact, it's fine if he becomes completely flaccid.

If your partner slips out of you in a flaccid state, lie on your back and have your partner lie on his side facing you. Place one of your legs on top of his and the other between his legs. Spread the opening of your vagina with your fingers and help your partner "stuff" his penis into you, from the base up, using two of his fingers as a splint.

Remember, the purpose of this exercise is not to become aroused to climax. The purpose of this exercise is simply to be still and be with your partner in this quiet, intimate, connected way.

DUTY-FREE INTERCOURSE

If you and your partner are used to approaching intercourse as a supersonic transport to orgasm, it's probably been a while since you allowed yourselves the luxury of a slow, languid screw, with no particular goal in mind except to enjoy the ride. Intercourse has become a means to an end, as opposed to a worthwhile journey in its own right. And that's where "duty-free" intercourse comes in.

Duty-free intercourse is about having no pressure, no destination, no expectations, and *no orgasms* (at least not intentionally). It is about rediscovering all of the possibility for sensation and connection inherent in the act of intercourse. It is about becoming more flexible and broaden-

ing your definition of what intercourse is, and
what it can be. Duty-free intercourse makes it easier to be in the moment instead of thinking ahead.

"Loving" Exercise #2

*To begin, you will take the active role (the one who is con-
trolling all of the movement) and your partner will take a
nonactive role; later, you will switch roles.*

*Kiss, hug, stroke, and fondle one another as you nor-
mally do when you make love. Give your partner a few genital kisses for good measure. When your partner is erect,
straddle him with your thighs and slide down on his penis.
Use lubricant if you like. Move up and down, round and
round, and side to side on your lover's penis. Move for your
own pleasure. But while you are moving any way you
want, it is very important that your partner's movements
are minimal. He needs to remain passive and just be "the
penis" that is there for your pleasure.*

*Since you both know you are not building toward
orgasm, your attention will stay on the sensation your
movement is creating for both of you. Be sure to LOOK at
your partner from time to time; having eye contact when
you make love will vastly increase your sense of connection
with your partner.*

*Switch positions and switch roles. Lie on your back as
your partner enters you. Your partner will stroke you, moving for his own pleasure, any way he wishes, just as you
did. Your movements should be minimal. And remember,
no orgasms allowed.*

How is intercourse different when you aren't focusing on having an orgasm and are left to focus solely on your genital connection? How are your partner's movements different? How are yours? How is his arousal different? How is yours?

When you have finished with your duty-free intercourse, hold each other and feel the energy coursing between you. This is energy that you can tap into whenever you want to by agreeing to have duty-free sex from time to time.

HEART TO HEART

Part of what makes great sex exciting is connecting with the rhythm of your partner as your level of excitement grows. And one of the best ways to connect with each other's rhythms is by listening to each other's heartbeats while you make love. Heart-to-heart intercourse creates a bridge and forms an incredible bond between you and your partner. It is an especially intense experience if one or both of you has an orgasm.

"Loving" Exercise #3
Using your hands and/or mouth, stimulate your partner until his penis is erect. Once he is erect, straddle him in the same way you did for duty-free sex. Begin moving sensuously on your partner's penis. As your arousal starts to build, lean over and place your right ear on the left side of your

partner's chest. Listen to his heart. How fast is it beating? Increase the speed and intensity of your thrusts. Does his heartbeat keep pace? Isn't it exciting to hear the physical evidence of your effect on your partner's arousal? Listening to your lover's heart during intercourse makes the experience more real. It will awaken you to the rhythms of your bodies, your arousal patterns, and, ultimately, each other.

Now it is his turn to be the active partner. For this exercise it is best for your partner to enter you from a kneeling position, between your legs, with his knees supporting most of his weight. If this position is awkward for either of you, place as many pillows as you need to underneath your buttocks to raise yourself up. Your partner is to begin slowly and sensuously thrusting. After a minute or two, he should lean over and place his ear on your heart. How many beats can he count in half a minute? Encourage him now to thrust more vigorously. Can he hear your heartbeat reflect your increased passion? Are you breathing more heavily?

Your partner should experiment with speeding up and slowing down his thrusts, listening to how it affects the beat of your heart. Once he has had a full listening experience, ask him to shift his body so that he can lie with his heart directly on top of yours; feel your hearts beating together as he thrusts to climax.

I AM YOU AND YOU ARE ME

Have you ever tried to imagine what your partner was physically feeling as you were making love?

This next exercise is often called "mutuality inter-course" because its goal is for both of you to pro-ject your awareness into each other's bodies dur-ing intercourse. By projecting your awareness and trying to feel what your partner is feeling, the physical boundaries separating the two of you are blurred, creating the sensation of merging with your partner. Mutuality intercourse is a very uni-fying experience and will leave you with the sense that the two of you together are greater than the sum of your parts.

"Loving" Exercise #4

You can make love in any position you like for this exercise. The important thing is to wait until you are both very aroused (through manual and/or oral stimulation) before initiating intercourse.

*Once intercourse begins, try to **experience** the intercourse through the sex organ of your partner: The woman should shift her awareness into her partner's penis and the man should shift his awareness into his partner's vagina. As she is being penetrated, the woman should ask herself, "Am I feeling my vagina or his penis?" The man should be asking himself, "Am I feeling my penis or her vagina?" What is "his" or "hers" becomes harder to discern; eventually, it will simply feel like "ours."*

The second variation of this exercise involves pretending that your physical positions are reversed. If you are on top, imagine that you are actually on the bottom. If you are the partner on the bottom, imagine that you are on top. This will also switch your focus from being the one who is thrusting to being the one thrusted into and vice versa. As you have intercourse and you both mutually switch focus in this way, you are likely to share the sensation that the two of you are holding on to each other and spinning or whirling through space. Slightly dizzying, yes, but also blissful.

A third variation to try is to place your consciousness into the entire body of your partner during intercourse and imagine experiencing the sex act with his or her **entire** body. What sensations is your partner experiencing? What smells? What tastes? What does the body contact feel like? What does it feel like for him to be on top of you or under you? What does it feel like for her to be under or on top? What does it feel like to penetrate you? What does it feel like to be penetrated by you? Feel a circle of energy surround and hold you both as you fully transfer your awareness into one another.

EVERY BREATH YOU TAKE

Breath is the stuff of life. And when you exchange breath with your partner, as you will soon learn to do, you experience his/her very life essence. The simple act of exchanging breath is a very loving and stimulating exercise. But combine breath exchange with intercourse and you have the makings of a sexual experience unlike any you have ever had.

"Loving" Exercise #5

The male partner will take the active role first in this exercise. After stimulating you with sensual caresses and kisses, your partner should position himself over you so that you are face-to-face. In the kneeling position described in "Loving" Exercise #3 (in between your legs, his weight supported by his knees), he will enter you and begin slow thrusting. As he continues to thrust back and forth, your partner should lean over and BREATHE into your mouth, one breath after the next. As he breathes into you, both of you should visualize his breath as a golden light entering your lungs, your stomach, your groin, passing through your vagina and back into him through his penis and up his spine. This creates a tremendous energy circle you both can feel. Continue breathing and thrusting for at least five full minutes.

When it is the woman's turn to take the active role (the role of "the breather"), stimulate your partner with sensual caresses and kisses to full or partial erection. Climb on top of him and slide his penis into your vagina. Begin moving sensuously up and down on his shaft. Continue thrusting as you lean over and begin breathing into his mouth. You will both visualize the breath as a ribbon of golden light that enters your lover's throat, moves down his esophagus and into his lungs, his abdomen, his pelvic area, entering his penis and coming back into you through your vagina and up your spine. Let the golden light fill you both until you feel it radiating out of you, encircling you in a golden cloud.

Sometimes the nonactive partner will find that he/she is approaching climax from the stimulation. If you are on the verge of climax, ask your partner to breathe one last breath into your mouth. Inhale deeply as you go over the brink into orgasm. Feel the warmth and energy of your lover's breath caress you from the inside as the delightful spasms overtake your body. After climaxing, lie on your side and draw your legs up slightly to form a modified "S" shape. Let your part-ner assume the same "S" shape, lying directly behind you, so that his/her "S" is cozied up to yours. Feel the breath going into and out of your bodies; nurture the connection you have created.

SEEING IS BELIEVING

Most of us close our eyes when we make love, par-ticularly when we are approaching climax. Though this seems like the "natural" thing to do, it is also a very effective way of cutting off the intensity of your connection. And that's not good! In this final lovemaking exercise, you are going to let your lover see your deepest passion and feel your vulnerability by gazing steadily into his eyes *the entire time* you are making love. Using this "eyes wide open" tech-nique, you will allow the phenomenal power that is transmitted through your eyes to seduce your part-ner all the way through the act of lovemaking, and magnify your sense of connectedness. I sometimes used this technique when I was a surrogate working with clients who had a particularly hard time staying centered and present: It made me feel like Svengali!

Now you may be wondering why I'm still talking about seduction at this late date. After all, you've already "gotten" one another, and you *are* already making love. But that's exactly why it's important to find new ways to seduce and mesmerize each other: to keep your sexual connection vibrant and fresh. Your concentrated gaze will have a hypnotic effect on your partner, and it will draw him out of himself and into you in some remarkable ways.

"Loving" Exercise #6

Caress your partner as you both keep your eyes open and focused on each other. Gaze deeply into each other's eyes and allow all of the love and desire you feel to shine through. Maintaining eye contact the entire time, I want you to take the more active role by climbing on top of your lover and lowering yourself onto his penis. Continue to make eye contact as you begin to move up and down, letting his penis caress you as it moves in and out.

Draw your sexual energies together as they build. Keep your movements sensuous and compel your partner to look back at you with the power of the sexual energy you are creating. Imagine that you are projecting a beam of white light from your eyes to your lover's; let yourself get lost in the world that exists just between the two of you. If either of

you approach orgasm, fight the impulse to close your eyes.
Try to keep your eyes open while you come, and after.

A LASTING CONNECTION

Once you become familiar with these different
ways of making love, you will find yourself naturally integrating elements of each into your lovemaking on a regular basis. There is nothing so
exciting as coming to a dead halt in the middle
of a mounting crescendo of passionate thrusts
and just remaining still for seconds at a time. Or
creating a laser beam of visual intensity as you
lock eyes with your partner seconds before
orgasm and let him witness the ecstasy that you
feel when you come. Try placing your consciousness into your partner's sex organs as you're giving oral sex to him and watch how it transforms
the way you conduct the act. With these exercises at your disposal, there is no reason to feel
disconnected from your partner during intercourse ever again.

12

Climax

n many ways, this has been a book about energy. We have explored various ways of finding, building, amplifying, manipulating, and storing sexual energy. Climax is also about energy. Climax is the moment when all of the sexual energy you have been building and storing comes to a head and is *released* all at once, like a flood that flows to every nerve ending in your body. Energetically speaking, climax truly is *le déluge*.

Was it Newton who said, "For every action, there is an equal and opposite reaction"? If it was, I wouldn't be surprised to learn that this theory came to him after a night of exquisite lovemaking. What we *all* have discovered during some of our most ardent adventures—whether we are scientists, mathematicians, poets, or stay-at-home moms—is that the more energy you can build and store before climaxing, the bigger the climax, or release, will be.

Before I go any farther, I want to point out that

up until this point, this book has not focused very much on the subject of climax. You may have found this peculiar, particularly since orgasm is such a huge and gorgeous part of the sexual experience. But, as always, my choice has been very intentional. Why? Because I haven't wanted you or your partner to become so fixated on your climax that all of the energizing stages in between become secondary. And I continue to hope that this will never be the case for both of you.

But there is no denying that climax holds the potential for extreme pleasure and connection with your partner on a level that virtually nothing else can provide. Climax can be pure bliss. Climax can be unforgettable. Climax can rock the house. Under the proper circumstances, climax even has the power to heal.

Can you increase the frequency, duration, and intensity of your climaxes? Yes, yes, and yes. Having come this far in the program, you've probably already experienced an orgasm or two that differs from any you have had before. But there are certain steps that you and your partner can take to *insure* that your climactic releases are always as full, as complete, and as pleasurable as is possible.

As you read through this chapter, notice that it follows the same course as that of an actual orgasm. First, we will focus on exercises that

build up a tremendous amount of energy before climax. Next, we will turn to ways to increase the intensity and duration of the **release** itself. And finally, we will learn ways to make the feelings **linger** long after the climax has "come" and gone. Build. Release. Linger. Let these three words become your new mantra—the three crucial steps on your journey to the stars.

BUILDING YOUR OWN STAIRWAY TO HEAVEN

One of the most powerful ways I know of to stockpile and control sexual energy and arousal is through a technique I call "stair-mastering." You actually had your first introduction to this in Level I of this book when you experimented with peaking. In stair-mastering, your levels of arousal are defined by a stairway of ten steps, where the first step represents very little or no arousal, the fifth step represents a constant, low-level arousal, and the tenth and highest step represents climax. You may currently feel as though your levels of arousal are better represented by an elevator— something over which you have little real control. Sometimes you shoot straight to the top, making you light-headed and giving you no time to explore any of the floors in between; at other times you get stalled out as other people get on or off and you linger far too long on floors you never intended to visit.

Stair-mastering gives you back the controls. Once you learn to master the stairs, you will see how you can slow down your ascent to the tenth stair by MAINTAINING on a step, or, how you can boost your ascent up the stairway by CLIMBING when you feel you're stuck on one stair for too long.

AROUSED, AWARE, AND IN CONTROL

In order to become familiar with your various levels of arousal, you and your partner are going to use the genital caress to experience climbing the "arousal stairwell." You can conduct this exercise independently of each other, but I encourage you to try it lying side by side. In addition to learning important information about your arousal, this is a wonderful opportunity for your partner to learn more about the subtleties of his own arousal. But he shouldn't feel pressured to participate in that way, and it is perfectly fine if he chooses to do nothing more than keep his arm wrapped around you through the exercise and be a witness to your own pleasure.

"Climax" Exercise #1

Take several slow, sensual breaths to the count of five. Ask your partner to do the same thing. Relax and center yourself. Begin stroking your genitals in a slow, sensuous manner (if he chooses to, your partner should stroke his genitals in the same fashion). As your arousal intensifies, designate a stair number for each new level you climb to. Take your time; this is not a goal-oriented exercise, except to become aware of your own unique arousal stairwell. If you get distracted, gently direct your attention back to your touch.

Caress yourself for twenty minutes or so. About every five minutes, check in and determine what arousal stair you are on. Repeat this exercise until you can consistently climb to stairs six and seven.

CLIMBING EVERY MOUNTAIN

For this next exercise, you are going to use the genital caress to experience the *control* you can exercise over your arousal level. The idea here is to bring yourself up to a certain stair level, and then let your arousal subside (dropping it to a lower level). Again, you can conduct this exercise by yourself. But in the interests of fusion, I recommend practicing with your partner.

"Climax" Exercise #2

Breathe, relax, and center yourself as you did in the previous exercise. Begin your genital caress (your partner should begin his own self-caress, if he so chooses). Remain aware of each step you climb as you continue with slow, constant strokes. **When you reach the fourth step, stop your caress and let your arousal go back down to step three or two.** *Then, slowly begin your caress again and let your arousal climb to step five. When you reach the fifth step, stop and again let your arousal drop down a couple of steps. Continue this exercise for twenty minutes or so, each time climbing to a higher step.*

When you finally reach the tenth stair, you will experience a keen and perhaps even explosive climax, a reaction to the slow and methodical "stockpiling" of sexual energy you practiced by climbing up and down the "stairway to heaven."

So now you are able to identify when you are on the ten different steps that lead to orgasm, as well as climb them at will. Just one more exercise to go before you are a certified "stair master."

RIDING THE WAVE

Mastering the art of "maintaining" involves learning to "hang out" on a certain stair level for a while without dropping down to lower steps. The ability to create these arousal plateaus puts you even more in control of your arousal levels and the amount of sexual energy you can build up for a more intense release.

There are four different methods you can use to maintain your arousal at a particular level. These four methods are:

1. squeezing your PC MUSCLE

2. altering your BREATHING

3. changing the speed and/or intensity of PELVIC THRUSTING

4. switching your FOCUS

(Men, if you are actively participating in this exercise, you can find your PC muscle the same way your partner found hers: It's the muscle you use to squeeze off the flow while urinating. It is also the muscle that can make your penis nod *yes* when it is erect. As Ross Perot is so fond of saying, "Are you with me?")

In order to become familiar with the way these four maintaining techniques can work, you are going to try each of these methods as you climb higher and higher on your arousal steps.

"Climax" Exercise #3
....
Using a genital caress, stroke yourself until you are on level five of your arousal stairway. **While you continue to stroke yourself, SLOW YOUR BREATHING** *until*

your arousal falls back to level four. Once you have reached level four, QUICKEN YOUR BREATHING until you rise to level six.

When you climb to level six, SQUEEZE YOUR PC MUSCLE several times until your arousal drops one step lower. Don't stop stroking yourself as you squeeze your PC muscle.

To employ the third technique, THRUST YOUR PELVIS sensuously against your hand as you stroke yourself. Imagine that you are being penetrated by your partner (men, imagine you are doing the penetrating). Bring yourself up to the seventh step in this way. When you're on the seventh step, stop thrusting and let your arousal fall back down to the sixth.

Stroke your genitals to bring yourself to level eight (you are breathing hard and are very excited at this point). At level eight, SWITCH YOUR MENTAL FOCUS FROM YOUR GENITALS to another part of your body that is **not** being stimulated. Focus on the tip of your nose or the lobe of your ear, for example. Watch your arousal level drop down a couple of steps.

Now, try thrusting against your hand again to come up to the ninth step. Stop thrusting long enough to come down to eight. See if you can use rapid breathing to bring you all the way up to the tenth step, and orgasm.

If you regularly practice these four maintaining techniques during intercourse or masturbation, they will soon become second nature to you. In very little time you will find yourself using them in various combinations without consciously having to think about it. I believe that the use of arousal awareness and the acts of climbing and maintaining can help to restore, preserve, and protect your libido. Twenty minutes of climbing and maintaining the arousal staircase is all it takes for endorphins to be produced and released by your body. Even if you don't have a climax, you will be bathed in the spine-tingling pleasure of one of nature's greatest gifts.

BAIT AND SWITCH

Most people associate the phrase "bait and switch" with the somewhat underhanded retailing practice of luring customers into a store with an advertised special and then pushing them to buy a much more expensive product once they get there. You will find my version of bait and switch far more benign, not to mention *stimulating*.

The purpose of bait and switch is to make a smooth transition from the lessons learned through self-discovery into their practical application with your partner. Bait and switch creates a physiological and behavioral bridge between being able to climax while masturbating and being able to climax during intercourse.

"Climax" Exercise #4

Combine caressing, oral stimulation, and stroking to bring your partner to erection. When he is aroused, climb aboard and begin to masturbate with his penis as you have done in earlier exercises. Glide the head back and forth over your clitoris as you work your way up the arousal staircase. **Focus now on you, your own pleasure.** I promise you, your "selfishness" will be a gift to both of you.

Once you climb to the highest stairs, SWITCH to your own fingers to stimulate your clitoris. Now slide down on your partner's penis. Masturbate to climax using your fingers with your partner's penis nestled inside you. Notice the intensity of feeling that is created by climaxing with the added stimulation of your lover's penis inside you. Use this technique often enough and you'll find you need direct clitoral stimulation less and less to achieve orgasm during intercourse.

Here are a few variations on this exercise that are also worth trying:

1. Keeping everything else in the exercise the same, enlist your partner to use *his* fingers to stimulate you to orgasm.

2. Instead of using your fingers, use a vibrator or vibrating dildo to stimulate your clitoris.

3. Alternate your hand, his hand, the tip of his penis, and the vibrator to bring you to the top of the "stairs." Work yourself up to levels eight and nine several times before you crest at the tenth stair.

DO COME IN

How would you like to be able to climax immediately upon penetration by your partner? IT CAN HAPPEN. There is a misconception shared by men and women alike that women are more likely to climax during intercourse the longer it goes on. Actually, the opposite is usually true. If a woman is NOT aroused before penetration, no amount of intercourse is going to make her come. If a woman IS aroused before penetration, however, she will most likely climax within the first seven minutes of intercourse. And if a woman is HIGHLY aroused, she can have an orgasm *immediately* upon penetration by her partner. The secret to success lies in already being at the "top of the stairs" when penetration occurs. Let me show you.

"Climax" Exercise #5

You are going to spend fifteen to twenty minutes pleasuring yourself and slowly climbing the arousal stairs. You can use your partner's penis to massage your clitoris and your vaginal lips, you can use a vibrator and a dildo, and you can certainly use genital stroking and caressing to work your way up the staircase.

Use the principles of loving touch to keep yourself in the here and now: Focus on the sensations that are created by your touch instead of dwelling on whether you are or aren't going to climax upon penetration. If you are anxious or worry about the orgasm, it probably won't happen. Enjoy the feelings you are experiencing **now**; let yourself get lost in them.

If you are using your partner's penis to caress yourself, you may not need to stimulate him to erection. But if he isn't erect once you are at the top of the stairs, you will need to stroke and/or suck your partner to erection while sustaining your own arousal by using the arousal maintenance techniques.

Now relax your PC muscle and the muscles in your buttocks, pelvic region, and thighs. Start breathing more rapidly.

Put a generous amount of lubricant on your partner's penis.

Have your partner lie on his back and position yourself directly over him. Close your eyes. Keep up the rapid breathing and self-caressing. When you are on the brink of climaxing, **open your eyes, inhale through your mouth, and thrust down to the base of your lover's penis.** You will most likely have an orgasm—if not immediately, then within the first five strokes.

If after several attempts you find that you have difficulty climaxing on the first stroke of penetration, try bringing yourself up to the ninth step several times, instead of just

*once, before you thrust down on your partner's penis. This
should help you have an orgasm on the first stroke.*

*(You can also try this exercise with your partner on top.
His signal to enter you is the deep breath and your eyes
opening wide. He should then thrust swiftly and deeply.)*

Your PC muscle can also play a very pleasurable role in triggering climax at the first stroke.
You would begin the exercise in exactly the same
way as described above. The twist comes at the
moment of penetration. Along with opening your
eyes and taking a deep breath, **clamp down
hard on your partner's penis with your PC
muscle as he enters you.** Spasm city!

CHAIN, CHAIN, CHAIN

Let's talk a little bit about multiple orgasms. I
first considered calling this section on multiple
orgasms "Skipping Stones," but I decided against
it because the circles created by a skipping stone
get smaller and smaller. This is sometimes the
case with multiple orgasms, but often the energy
that is released remains constant, or even grows
in intensity. So instead of a skipping stone on the
surface of a pond, I will paint a picture of links in
chains of various shapes and sizes, with no two
chains ever being exactly alike.

Any position can lend itself to your having a string of orgasms: man on top, woman on top, front to back, or on all fours. Initially, you may find that being on top gives you the most access, flexibility, and control. But choose a position that works best for you. Or better yet, choose them all! Different positions may produce different kinds of orgasms; some may feel more clitoral and others more vaginally inspired.

Before you attempt to have multiple orgasms with your partner, however, it may help if you first experiment with having them on your own. (Once you are able to experience multiple orgasms on your own, you will discover that it is much easier to incorporate the experience into lovemaking.) How are you going to do this? By using a combination of genital caresses and stimulation from a dildo or a vibrator to peak yourself to orgasm and *maintain* your arousal level on that fabulous tenth stair. This will continue the orgasmic chain. Practice this now.

When you have been able to stimulate a chain of orgasms in yourself at least two or three times, you are ready to try it with your partner. Remember that being able to let yourself go, stay out of your head, and surrender to the exquisite sensations being created in your body are what will most influence your ability to link your orgasms in one long, red-hot chain.

"Climax" Exercise #6

Once you and your partner are sufficiently aroused, "assume the position" (on your back, legs in the air, your partner kneeling between your legs) and begin having intercourse. Use clitoral stimulation during intercourse (fingers or vibrator) to climb to stairs four, five, and six. Maintain your arousal at level seven through breathing, pelvic thrusting, squeezing your PC, or switching your focus. Proceed up the stairs to levels eight and nine. Instead of maintaining there, as several other exercises have asked you to do, let yourself fall over the edge into orgasm. BUT DO NOT REST. CONTINUE STIMULATING YOURSELF UNTIL YOU CLIMAX AT LEAST ONE MORE TIME.

Guys, don't feel shortchanged. You too can learn to have multiple orgasms. It involves that all-important PC muscle again and you can read all about it in my book *How to Make Love All Night (and Drive a Woman Wild)*.

FAKE IT TILL YOU MAKE IT

As I near the end of this chapter, I realize that there may be some readers who are frustated because they have yet to have an orgasm with their partners. If you are one of those readers, I hope the next exercise will change that for you.

You may be surprised that I would encourage you to fake anything sexual, let alone orgasm! I can understand why you would be. Faking orgasm has earned *its* bad rap because it is equated with false flattery, deception, and guile. And guess what? It's not only women who practice it; studies have shown that men do it too! Now, I am not a fan of faking orgasm to please a partner; I believe everybody loses in that scenario. But what if instead of simulating orgasm to "fake" out your partner, you used orgasmic behavior to *encourage your body* into producing the real thing? *That* would be an orgasm worth faking!

Let me show you how this works. When you have a powerful orgasm, your face contorts, your back arches, you involuntarily cry out, you may experience spasms in your arms and legs, and your PC muscle contracts. In other words, you feel an orgasm all over your body, not just in your vagina. So when you are at a high enough peak on your arousal scale, by acting "as if"—by contorting your face, arching your back, crying out, spasming your arms and legs, and fluttering your PC muscle—you can often trigger an actual orgasm.

"Climax" Exercise #7

Once you and your partner are sufficiently aroused, begin intercourse. Choose a position where you feel you have the most control over your levels of arousal (some women will prefer to be on top of their partners for this exercise). Breathe deeply, relax, and focus on your physical sensations. Use pelvic thrusts, PC squeezes, and clitoral stimulation in addition to the thrusting motions of intercourse to get your blood flowing and heart racing. When you are at that place where you feel orgasm is imminent but usually doesn't arrive, first **take ten to fifteen rapid inhalations through your nose.** Then, AS SIMULTANEOUSLY AS YOU CAN MANAGE:

1. Take a deep breath.
2. Suck in your tummy.
3. Arch your back.
4. Open your eyes up *wide*.
5. Cry out (nothing fancy required; you just need to encourage the release of energy).
6. Relax your PC muscle (if you don't immediately climax, try pulsing your PC muscle a few times to activate it).

It's a lot of coordinating at first (if you are finding it difficult to coordinate all of these steps, try practicing one or two at a time as you climb and maintain at the higher arousal levels), but you may very well prompt a genuine orgasm. If you have never had an orgasm before and don't quite know what to be on the lookout for, you will experience it as an involuntary pulsating or spasming in your vagina. It isn't always huge, or earth-shattering, but it is always pleasurable.

(You may prefer to practice exhibiting the behaviors of orgasm by yourself before attempting it with your partner. If *you do, spend twenty minutes climbing and maintaining to first bring yourself to a highly aroused state. Then, proceed as outlined above.)*

Being fully sexually connected requires being honest with yourself and your partner. If you have trouble achieving orgasm when you have intercourse, you are neither less of a woman nor guilty of a crime. Let your partner know. Let him help you create an atmosphere of safety and support where you are free to relax, free to feel, and free to climax.

If this exercise helps you have your first orgasm with your partner, you will be flooded with intense emotion afterward. Even if you frequently have orgasms when you make love, using the climbing and maintaining techniques can elevate them to a whole new level of ardor for you. But we're not done yet. Coming up are some special ways to bond with your lover after you have "danced together at the top of the stairs."

GLOW ON

Between the lovemaking experiences that you had in the previous chapter and the orgasmic experiences you have had in this one, some doors may have opened in your heart that have led you to places of great love and communion with your partner. After an experience like that, the last thing you want to do is abruptly break the connection by lighting a cigarette, turning on the TV, or immediately falling asleep. An abrupt disconnection from your partner after this kind of intercourse can be a jarring experience. And it can rob you of most of the greatest payoffs you have been working toward.

If you keep the connection, on the other hand, your reward is often an intense emotional experience that is worthy of poetry. Close, connected, and intense sex opens us up and makes us feel extremely vulnerable. It is not unusual to laugh until you cry or cry until you laugh after an intense lovemaking session. Just as when we try to repress any one emotion it winds up repressing them all to a certain degree, when we release a tremendous amount of sexual energy it releases many other energies and emotions along with it—energies such as love, sadness, ecstasy, joy, or some combination of each. You need to honor those feelings as they come up and let them bring you closer to who you are and who you and your partner can be together.

One very simple way to "hold the moment" is to remain physically engaged for as long as possible after you have climaxed. Stay in each other's arms and let your partner's erection slowly subside while his penis remains inside you. Enjoy the lingering orgasmic sensations as your PC muscles periodically spasm and you both float back down to earth. Keeping your eyes open and gazing at each other maintains the sense of connection even more. Remain silent as you stroke one another's faces and look deeply into each other's eyes. Feel the glow.

TO HAVE AND TO HOLD

Here are more special "postcoital cuddles" for you and your loved one to try that will prolong the bonding power of your climax.

1. Spooning. Covered in an earlier chapter as well, this position usually finds the female partner with her back nestled up against her lover's chest, and both partners' knees drawn up slightly to form an "S" shape. The male partner can use his free arm to gently stroke his lover's body, or to simply hold her near. To feel really connected, synchronize your breaths. Naturally, the positions can be reversed.

2. The heart hug. Lie on your sides, facing each other. Look into each other's eyes. Whoever is going to receive the hug slides down until her/his ear is resting on his/her

partner's chest, near the heart. Listen to your lover's heart beat more and more slowly as he/she wraps his/her arms around you and you nestle against them.

3. The shoehorn. One partner sits up in bed, propped up with pillows, legs extended and slightly parted. The other partner slips in between his/her legs and lies back against the other's chest. The partner being cradled can use her/his fingertips to lightly stroke the other's legs.

TAKING TIME TO REFLECT

Take a moment to think back on who and where you were when you first started on the path to profound sexual connection. Can you believe you're the same person? In many ways, you are not the same at all. The risks you have taken have changed your understanding of yourself, your partner, and your capacity for pleasure. Both you and your partner are to be praised for having the courage and taking the time to build such a meaningful and rewarding connection.

In the final chapter of this book, you will discover exercises that will take you, along with your partner, to even more exotic sexual destinations—destinations you may not have even known existed. Grounded in a solid foundation of knowledge of each other's bodies, trust in each other's actions, and respect for each other's feelings, you are free to explore the farthest reaches of sexual expression together. While I hesitate to say that I've saved "the best" for last, I've certainly saved a lot. You've had an extraordinary meal—a sensual buffet. If you can find the room, it's time for a few bites of dessert.

13

Edges

You have to climb a lot of hills before you scale Mount Everest. You have to scramble a lot of eggs before you attempt a soufflé. And you have to have a strong and vital connection to your partner at the heart of your sexual relationship before venturing out to your sexual edges.

Perhaps you feel that this book has already brought you to, or perhaps even slightly beyond, what you imagine to be your sexual edges and you are feeling completely content with your new sexual connection. If this is how you are feeling right now, you should feel free to stop here. You've already done a magnificent job, and you've done more than enough. Now is the time to fully enjoy it. You can always return to this chapter next month, next year, or whenever your curiosity surfaces. But if you're ready to "ice" the cake, and it doesn't feel like quittin' time yet, this is the chapter you've been waiting for.

By completing the previous exercises that were specifically designed to build your trust, increase intimacy, and broaden your knowledge of one another, you are in a position to reap maximum benefit from the exercises in this final chapter. The exercises you are about to encounter will carry you beyond the "normal" realm of lovemaking. And for this reason, I need to issue a very clear warning: Engaging in these exercises without first creating that safe, close, and loving context will feel, at best, hollow, and, at worst, extremely isolating. Intimacy, familiarity, and acceptance are the necessary ingredients that turn what may at first glance look like "kinky" exercises into vehicles for unimaginable pleasure between a loving couple, as well as being the ultimate expression of the love and trust two people can share. But the intimacy must come first. These exercises are not intended as a substitute for intimacy, nor as a means to avoid it.

WHERE ARE YOUR EDGES?

Because I am a sex therapist who has been educated through literally thousands of sessions with clients over the years, I am comfortable making a few general assumptions about where your sexual edges may lie. But the truth of the

matter is, women's and men's sexual edges come
in as many variations as the people themselves.
What one woman might consider to be her
wildest sexual fantasy may fall into the "been
there, done that" category for someone else. No
one (not even the most experienced sex therapist) can fully define your edges for you except
y-o-u.

So where do *your* sexual edges lie? Do you
know? Where are you still saying no to yourself?
What are the sexual fantasies you have that still
make you feel uncomfortable? What are the sexual fantasies you have that you can't quite turn
into reality? What are the sexual fantasies you
have that you struggle to embrace, even in your
own mind?

It's time to integrate this missing piece of yourself and form the complete, fully sexual you. To
surrender means to accept, remember? To surrender to the connection means to *accept* every
aspect of yourself—even the aspects you might
have dismissed until this day as unacceptable,
weird, or politically incorrect. As long as your
edges don't involve injury or harm to yourself,
your partner, or your relationship, they should be
embraced and celebrated as aspects of your won-
derfully alive and creative sexual nature. They
should not fill you with fear, they should fill you

with fascination. And they can also fill you with new and exciting erotic opportunity.

IS THAT REALLY ME?

Before you can embrace your sexual edges, you must first locate these edges. If you've been repressing your edgiest sexual urges for a long time, you may not have them at your fingertips, and a little "excavating" may be called for in order to unearth them. As I said before, I can't tell you exactly what your edges are. But what I can do is give you pathways to discovering these edges for yourself, pathways born of years of experience. And that brings us to our first exercise.

This is the only time in this chapter I am going to ask you and your partner to complete an exercise independently of one another. You can both do the exercise at the same time, but you each need your own private space. This may feel contrary to the concept of "fusion." But in order to be perfectly candid with yourself in the process of locating your edges, you must feel completely safe and free from judgment of any kind. And that includes the judgments of the one you love. When the exercise has been completed, you can come together and reconnect by talking about the experience. Trust that the material generated from completing this exercise will create many opportunities for enhancing your connection.

"Edges" Exercise #1

You should each choose a comfortable spot where you can sit undisturbed. Have a pad of paper nearby and something to write with. At the top of the page, write:

A SEXUAL FANTASY OF MINE THAT MAKES ME FEEL
VERY GUILTY OR UNCOMFORTABLE IS:

Think about your answer but don't write anything else yet. First close your eyes, breathe deeply into your stomach, and relax. Now allow the fantasy to surface in your mind's eye. Let it play out without interruption and without censorship. Make yourself a "fly on the wall," so to speak, and simply observe the action. Be aware of what you are feeling. Are you aroused? Uncomfortable? A little or a lot of both? Do you feel like masturbating? Go ahead. Bring yourself to orgasm if you want to. When the fantasy has ended, continue to breathe deeply. Slowly open your eyes and reach for your pad.

In your journal, finish the sentence you started at the top of the page. Describe the fantasy in full detail. Write down all of the elements of the fantasy you just had. Be sure to include:

- *who was involved*
- *where it took place*
- *the time of day, the setting, the mood*

- *what was worn by whom*
- *what was said and who said it*
- *who did what to whom*
- *if there were any props, accessories, or inanimate objects involved*
- *anything else you can remember regarding what happened in the fantasy*

Be an objective reporter. Judgmental words about what you did in the fantasy are not allowed. When you have described the fantasy as completely as possible, turn to a fresh page and write at the top:

THE WAY THIS FANTASY MAKES ME FEEL IS:

*Now write down **all** of the feelings that came up or are still coming up for you regarding this fantasy. Don't leave anything out. Talk about your excitement, your guilt, your discomfort, your fear . . . whatever feelings you may have.*

Do you have other fantasies that also make you feel guilty or slightly uncomfortable? Feel free to "wander through" some of these fantasies right now, one by one. Try to write about at least one or two more in your journal. And return to this exercise when others come to mind.

WRESTLING WITH PAPER TIGERS

Once you have written down your fantasies and feelings, I want you to ask yourself these three questions:

1. *Where are you right now?*
   I'm not speaking figuratively, I mean literally. Where are you? Are you anywhere
   you aren't supposed to be? Aren't you
   still safe at home, sitting on your bed or
   in an armchair the same way you would
   be if you were watching TV? I believe you
   are. So your fantasy doesn't have the
   power to physically transport you somewhere else.

2. *Who is with you right now?*
   You're still by yourself, right? No one
   (including your partner) suddenly material-
   ized beside you dressed in the outfit you
   fantasized them in, doing the things you
   fantasized them doing, did they? Of course
   not. So your fantasy doesn't have the
   power to make people materialize either.

3. *Has your love for your partner changed?*
   Are your feelings for your partner the
   same now as before you had the fantasy?
   Are you planning to remain with him,
   love and cherish him as you always have?
   You are? Then that must mean that your
   fantasy doesn't have the power to alter
   your feelings for or commitment to your
   partner either.

I'm not trying to be critical or clever. I'm trying to help you see that even your edgiest fantasies actually have very little power. So why do
you feel so bad about them? Just because you
have a fantasy doesn't mean you have an obliga-
tion to make it come true. Even more important:
YOUR FANTASIES DO NOT HAVE THE
POWER TO AFFECT REALITY *UNLESS*
THAT IS WHAT YOU WANT. You don't have
to act them out unless that is what you want.
You don't have to share them with anyone unless
that is what you want. But your fantasies *are* a
part of who you are. And that is a reality that
will never change. There is no reason to deny
that reality. It is not healthy for you to deny that
reality. You need to embrace it, and to embrace
those edges. Even if the only embracing is hap-
pening in your mind.

Everyone has sexual fantasies. And many of
these fantasies are probably far more "edgy" and
outrageous than yours. People can get aroused
at the strangest times and by the strangest
things. I know a happily married mother of two
beautiful children who gets incredibly aroused at
funerals. Does she act out in inappropriate
ways? Only in her mind. Does she feel the need
to make an announcement about her sudden
surge of desire? No, she does not. But she doesn't
go around beating herself up about it either. It is

what it is. It is not harmful to anyone. And she accepts that. By accepting *your* sexual edges wholeheartedly and without shame, you may find that the energy that it took to stay away from them is freed to fuel your sexual engine to an even greater degree.

I am not going to ask you to show or discuss the fantasies you have been writing about with your partner. In fact, I suggest that both of you destroy the written portion of this exercise in order to protect your privacy. If you want to discuss your fantasies or the possibility of acting out portions of them with your partner, that's fine. And you'll have many opportunities in this chapter to experiment with all kinds of fantasies. But as far as I am concerned, you are also allowed to have fantasies that you keep to yourself. These are some of *your edges*. You share them or don't share them only as *you* choose. The important thing is that you don't hide them from *yourself*.

WAKING THE SLEEPING BEAUTY

It's time to start tiptoeing in the direction of your sexual edges hand in hand with your loving partner. This next exercise, which I call "Sleeping Beauty," is an exercise that simply would not be possible between a couple who did not know each other well, and trust each other implicitly (if you have *any* doubts, stop now). Playing Sleeping Beauty continues to build on that trust; it also gives both of you a hiatus from performance pressure of any kind.

"Edges" Exercise #2

*To begin this exercise, one partner (the "sleeping beauty") lies motionless, as though asleep. You can start fully clothed. The other partner (the active partner) then drapes a towel or light cloth over the passive partner's face. For the next thirty minutes, the active partner treats the inactive partner like a love toy and gets to pleasure herself/himself on **any** part of the sleeping partner's body in **any** way he/she pleases.*

The sleeping partner does not move, does not speak, and does not respond (except, of course, for involuntary responses like erections, natural lubrication, and orgasm!). Make sure there is plenty of lubricant on hand, and that it is used generously, wherever appropriate. Please note: If anything hurts you or makes you uncomfortable, you should always feel free to speak up immediately.

As the active partner, take note of the way you are behaving. How is it different from the way you usually conduct yourself with your partner when you are having sex? Are you less gentle? Less "politically correct"? Is your partner getting aroused? What does that tell you about the effect your pleasing yourself has on him/her? As the passive part-

ner, take note of how you're feeling, too. Are you more
relaxed or less relaxed than usual? More aroused or less
aroused? Does it excite you to fully give up control? If you
experience any anxiety while playing Sleeping Beauty,
repeating the exercise several times will help you develop the
level of trust you need to fully relax and enjoy yourself.

Switch roles after thirty minutes. When the exercise is
complete, choose a cuddling position in which to hold each
other and talk about the experience you just shared.

SOMETIMES YOU WANT TO BE A SLAVE TO LOVE

Remember playing Three Questions ("Asking"
Exercise #4) with your partner earlier in this
program? This next exercise, which I call "Love
Slave," is the graduate-level version of that exercise from Chapter 9. As in Three Questions, one
partner controls the actions of the other partner.
But that's where the similarities end.

Love Slave turns the concept of asking for
what you want on its head. Because this time
you don't have to ask nicely. You're the boss. You
tell your partner what to do because you are the
master and your partner is your love slave. For
this one exercise, it's okay if your requests do
sound like demands. And you get to demand
whatever you want, however many times you

want it, during your thirty-minute turn. But before you lose your mind completely, note that your partner *always* has the right to refuse anything unreasonable. But it has to be unreasonable. Simply being "not in the mood" is not a good reason to have your requests denied. If you or your partner are not "in the mood" to touch a few edges, you shouldn't be doing the exercise.

"Edges" Exercise #3

The exercise begins the minute you close the bedroom door. You can start by telling your partner what kind of music you want to hear, how you want the lights adjusted, if you want candles to be lit, etc. The love slave is to obey, while remaining absolutely **silent**. *Once the mood has been set to your satisfaction, you want to tell your love slave what clothing to put on or take off, what toys to bring to bed, where to sit, stand, or lie down—whatever you like. Maybe you want to be fanned. Maybe you want to be fed peeled grapes. Maybe you want to be massaged with hot oil. The decisions are all yours. What's next? Maybe you want to be teased. Maybe you want to be penetrated. Maybe you want to masturbate while your partner does nothing but watch. Unless there is a serious objection to an order, the love slave remains silent, compliant, and obedient throughout the exercise while carrying out his or her "master's" wishes.*

But listen up: Be careful not to abuse your power. This exercise is not an excuse for you to be sadistic or heavy-

handed. There is absolutely no yelling and no reprimanding allowed. You both have an opportunity while in the "master" role to gain even more of your partner's trust; be sure to earn it.

*If you tend to be the more dominant sexual partner in your relationship, how does it feel to have no control? If you tend to be the more passive sexual partner, how does it feel to have **all** the control? Whether you are playing the master or playing the love slave, this exercise can be a big-time turn-on for both partners if you feel comfortable enough with yourselves and with each other; how is it for you?*

After each of you has had a turn in both roles, get into a cuddling position. Talk about the thoughts and feelings that came up for you in each role. Did you enjoy it? Would you do it again? Hold each other gently until you feel satisfied you have shared everything you need to.

As are all of the exercises I have designed for loving couples, playing master and slave is meant to break down barriers between you, heighten your sense of intimacy, and increase your self-awareness. If ever you feel the opposite is occurring during an exercise, stop, and talk about it immediately.

MUTUAL ORAL STIMULATION

Commonly referred to as "69," mutual oral stimulation (MOS) is a position that many people talk about. But I wonder how many of those people have ever actually tried it and are familiar with the exquisite pleasures it can provide? One of the reasons MOS is so arousing is because it naturally encourages each partner to constantly switch focus; one moment your attention is on the pleasure you are giving, the next moment it's on the pleasure you are receiving. Continuously switching focus in this way forces each partner to spontaneously climb and maintain on "the stairs" of arousal, stockpiling energy as you go.

Another reason MOS is so exciting is because it is such a comprehensive way to *physically* connect. Two warm, loving mouths connecting to two sensitive sets of genitals, with both partners actively giving *and* receiving pleasure. Wow.

Have *you* ever tried MOS? If you haven't, you're about to find out what you've been missing. If you *are* familiar with its delights, stick around; there's something new for you to try, too.

"Edges" Exercise #4

MOS works best with the woman on top, or with both partners on their sides, head to feet. Start with a slow, oral caress. Use your tongue to explore your partner's genitals; feel the textures of the skin, the ridges and the folds. For the first thirty seconds, focus on the sensation of giving pleasure to your partner. After thirty seconds, switch your focus to the sensations your partner is giving you. Move your hips, moan, and let yourself get lost in the pleasure. After another thirty seconds, switch your focus back to what you are doing. Begin to increase the speed and intensity with which you caress your partner. Switch focus again after thirty more seconds. Continue to build and climb in this fashion.

Since both of you are switching focus at thirty-second intervals and increasing your intensity at the same pace, it is possible that you will bring each other to climax simultaneously, or nearly so. The combination of experiencing your partner's orgasm so directly while you yourself are in the throes of intense sexual passion will forge a particularly powerful bond.

Here's another variation on mutual oral gratification for the adventurous edge explorer.

"Edges" Exercise #5

Have a penis-sized dildo and a butterfly vibrator on hand before you begin. Engage in the MOS exercise as described above. After a minute or two, the female partner should raise herself several inches over her lover's face by resting on her knees; her top half remains lowered over his torso and groin. Men, insert the dildo into your lover and begin to slide it in and out of her vagina while you continue to give her oral pleasure.

The female partner straps the butterfly vibrator onto the back of her hand and holds the base of her lover's penis with that hand while she continues to orally stimulate him. The vibrations from the dildo will travel through your hand to gently stimulate your lover's penis and testicles.

As in the previous exercise, both partners should continue to shift focus every thirty seconds as they erotically build toward climax.

TIE ME UP, TIE ME DOWN

We've all seen those movies where some poor, unsuspecting guy lets himself be tied up by a bewitching vixen only to find out that she's really a thief or a lunatic who leaves him to be discovered later in this very compromising position. Or those movies where the innocent heroine is tied to the bed by a love-obsessed stranger. But this isn't the movies. And the beauty of exploring bondage with your loving partner is that you don't have to worry about any of that crazy stuff! Does that make "playful bondage" boring? Not a chance. Even with a loving partner, there remains a slightly "dangerous" element to the act of bondage, and that element is one of the things that makes tying your partner up, or being tied up by your partner, edgy and exciting.

This is another exercise that should only be engaged in by the most secure and loving couples. It is your sensitivity to your partner, coupled with the good communication skills that you have, that will make your experience with playful bondage an erotic adventure in the world of sexual connection instead of an exercise in frustration.

"Edges" Exercise #6

Use nylons (my personal favorite), silky scarves, or restraints purchased at an adult store to gently tie your lover to the bed or to a comfortable chair. It is up to both of you to decide what part or parts of the body you will restrain: arms or legs . . . or both? Obviously, it is important that the partner being tied up (passive partner) is comfortable in every respect. The passive partner has no responsibility at all in this exercise except to remain aware of his/her own feelings and sensations.

Once the tied-up partner is comfortable, the active partner can proceed to pleasure herself (himself) with her (his) lover's body. As the active partner, you can rub up against, lick, suck, probe, and sit on your partner, as long as you are not making them uncomfortable and they do not object for any reason.

Are you having any new sensations as you ravage your restrained mate? Any new impulses or fantasies? And what about you, the tied-up partner? Are you feeling sexy? Have you let go of every last modicum of reserve? When you have trust in your partner and in yourself, you feel free to experience all of the feelings your sexuality arouses in you.

For this exercise, I don't recommend trading places in the same evening. One thirty- to forty-minute session using restraints is usually enough for one night. Don't get me wrong. You both deserve a turn being tied, or doing the tying. But bondage can be an intense experience for both participants and you may want to wait a day or two before reversing the roles. Let the feelings linger.

Here are two variations on a theme of playful bondage that you might not want to miss.

"Edges" Exercise #7
Begin the exercise as you did in "Edges" Exercise #6. Once your partner has been tied up, use a long feather to play with your lover's body. Starting at the top of the head, slowly run the feather down the length of your lover's body, stopping at the nipples, the belly button, and the genitals, of course.

*If your partner is agreeable to it, place a **blindfold** over his/her eyes. Keep it there as you use the feather to caress them, and later, as you make love to them.*

I have received an endless stream of glowing reports from my clients who try the dynamic duo of restraints and blindfold. Many of my female clients in particular count it as one of the most erotic experiences of their lives. As long as we're giving testimonials, I have to admit that it has rated off the charts for me as well. It may be a little bit out on the edge, but it does wonders for your feeling of sexual connection.

DINNER FOR TWO,
WITH NO RESERVATIONS

Why does dinner by candlelight always seem to lead to sex? Why does dinner under the stars always seem to lead to sex? Why does dinner at your favorite restaurant always seem to lead to sex? Let's face it, food and sex just go together. So why resist the natural connection? Instead, why not *amplify* that connection and take it to its edges?

In the following exercise, plates disappear, utensils disappear, perfect manners disappear and Emily Post takes a holiday. It's your first orgy, an orgy for two, and all you need is mountains of food. So assemble all of your favorite finger foods—that's anything you can eat with your hands—and spare no expense if you can. Canapés and caviar, soft cheese and fruits (the juicier, the better), pâtés and mousses, chicken and ribs and any other meats that can be pulled off the bone. If it makes a mess, it's the kind of food you want, especially if it's a mess you can lick off your fingers. Focus on soft foods that feel particularly sensuous in the mouth. Get some bottled beverages to complement your feast—champagne or wine or fruit juice or sparkling water, depending on whether or not you drink alcohol. Now find an old blanket, an old sheet, or several large towels that you aren't afraid to soil, find your partner, and let the exercise begin.

"Edges" Exercise #8

Spread your blanket (or sheet or towels) on the floor to protect your carpet and furniture. Dim the lights, light a few candles nearby, play some soft music, and take off all of your clothing. Relax now with your partner. Caress each other. Take several slow, sensuous breaths, and prepare to begin your feast.

There are three rules for this special dinner: 1) no talking; 2) no utensils; 3) you cannot feed yourself.

So begin now, feeding each other. And focus on the delicious experience of every morsel of food as it passes from your lover's fingers to your eager lips. Chew slowly. Immerse yourself in the moment. Watch your partner as you fill his/her mouth with pleasure.

Drink from the bottle. Don't be afraid to spill. Be reckless with your food and lick your "accidents" off each other's bodies. You may feel the urge to have sex right in the middle of this wild dinner for two. Don't fight it. Surrender to the momentary madness and thrash about making even more of a mess. When you are done, you can wash each other off with warm, wet towels or take a sensuous shower together.

WITH A CHERRY ON TOP

At the end of the last chapter, I asked if you had any room left for dessert, and you probably thought I was speaking figuratively. But, as you're about to discover, I'm a very literal person! And it's time for your just desserts.

I wanted your last exercise in the book to be playful, sensual, fun, and *delicious*. Nothing quite meets all of those criteria the way ice cream does; an ice cream *sundae,* to be exact. You've probably made your own sundae at the local ice cream parlor before. The difference is that this time when you lick the dish clean, your "dish" may writhe, giggle, or moan, because you will be giving someone very close to you an exquisite "tongue-lashing."

You will need to assemble the following ingredients:

- ice cream (slightly softened, not rock hard)
- chocolate, caramel, butterscotch, marshmallow, and/or pineapple sauce (at room temperature)
- maraschino cherries and banana slices
- whipped cream (now available fat free!)
- sprinkles

To fully experience the subtle nuances that come with being either the sundae or the sundae maker, I suggest you take turns in both roles (instead of both of you becoming sundaes at the same time).

"Edges" Exercise #9

It's time to make your own sundaes. To begin, take a sensuous shower or bath together. Gently wash each other's backs, legs, and genitals. Rinse off completely and towel dry. Set a mood for yourselves: Light some candles, play music, burn incense; breathe, relax, and slow down. Sit down in the tub together. Have your sundae makings within easy reach.

Start your sundae with one of your sauces. (The sauces can be warmed *ever so slightly* in a saucepan or micro-wave oven before you begin the exercise; just make sure to check carefully that they're not too hot before you apply them.) Pour some of your sauce onto your lover's chest. Then take your hands and slowly massage the sauce over the surface of his/her skin. Luxuriate in the thick, warm texture of the sauce beneath your fingers. Lick the sauce from your lover's nipples. See how it tastes off other parts of his/her anatomy, as well. Now add some ice cream. The chill will be slightly shocking, but it will also be pleasant and very stimulating. Slowly massage the ice cream all over your lover's body; lick some of it off the most sensitive spots.

Add a layer of whipped cream. Be generous in your application so you can really play with its fluffy consistency. Use the whipped cream as a lubricant as your hand glides up and down your lover's penis, or strokes her vagina. Finish off your sundae with bananas, sprinkles, and a cherry on top. Now lick your lover clean.

Switch roles and let the sundae become the sundae maker. After you have had a turn in both roles, put all of the leftovers into the tub with you and "smush" your bodies together. Revel in the slippery, slidy, gooey, velvetiness of it all and in the joyous freedom you have achieved with your partner.

AND SOME TO GROW ON

How are you feeling right now? Do you feel like you've done all of the "edge exploration" you can handle for one lifetime? Or did the lyrics to "We've Only Just Begun" suddenly pop into your head? If you are among those who are grateful to have revived a sense of adventure, trust, and playfulness in your sexual relationship with your partner, but who need to take a breather from the "outer limits" of lovemaking, now would definitely be the time. You have done great work. You have embraced this adventure. And the rewards are already evident in the new connections you have made with yourself, and the connections you have made with your loving partner.

On the other hand, if you are a dedicated "wing walker" and your appetite has merely been whetted for the new and completely different, don't let me be the one to stop you. There are so many more edges for you to explore. Maybe you're ready to take your partner with you on another "blue" shopping spree. That'll give you a few new ideas, not to mention a shopping cart full of new props to help set the stage. Or maybe it's time for a completely sexual weekend—two days and nights dedicated to nothing but sexual experimentation with the one you love—at a hotel or motel where you are far from prying eyes. Perhaps you're ready to learn about the delights of some playful spanking, or ready to play the part of the "stern mistress of discipline." How about holding your "First Annual Erotic Film Festival for Two" in the privacy of your own bedroom? These are just a few of the edges you've yet to explore.

Edges are something that only you and your partner can fully define. Nothing is weird unless it's weird for *you*. Nothing is wrong unless it's wrong for *you*. And nothing is too much unless it's too much for *you*. Let your instincts, impulses, and inspirations be your guide. There is only one thing I ask of you: Always remember that your number one priority is to strengthen and maintain the *connection*.

CONNECTED AT LAST

Think back to who you were before you began this program: Can you imagine that person engaging in some of the exercises you have now completed? Could you *ever* have imagined sharing some of the experiences you now have had with your partner before you committed to the program of getting close and connected? *You* may be surprised, but I'm not; the minute you bought this book and brought it home, I knew you had it in you. You had the *will* and so you *paved the way* for a new level of open, loving, sexual expression with yourself and with your partner.

Your sexual connection is an ongoing process. The foundations of your connection—loving touch, visualization, writing, PC muscle squeezes, and all of the other building blocks you developed along the way—are the touchstones you will return to time and time again. Incorporating these basics into your regular routine will help keep your connection alive, vital, and crackling with energy.

For me, life is about living healthfully, loving deeply, and laughing as often as I can. I hope I have helped you live a little more "out loud" and that you will renew your commitment to being a fully sexually connected woman and having a close, sexually connected partnership every single day of your life.

Appendix:
Toys

*t*he following is a list of popular companies that sell dildos, vibrators, and other sex toys through the mail and on-line (via the Internet). While I do not feel comfortable personally endorsing any of these companies, I have conducted trouble-free business with all of them. Call or write for catalogs, or contact them at their Web sites.

Good Vibrations
San Francisco, CA
1-415-974-8990
http://www.goodvibes.com

Intimate Treasures
San Francisco, CA
1-415-863-5002
http://www.intimatetreasures.com

Xandria Collection
Department C 1096
P.O. Box 31039
San Francisco, CA 94131-9988
http://www.xandria.com

Lady Calston
908 Niagara Falls Blvd., Suite 519
Lake Tonawanda, NY 14120-2060
1-800-690-5239
http://www.calston.com

Adam and Eve
P.O. Box 900
Department CS 357
Carrboro, NC 27510
1-800-274-0333
http://www.adameve.com